Living with Taiji

Resilience through Inner Power

by

Frieder Anders

with

Emanuel Seitz

Three Pines Press
St. Petersburg, FL 33713
www.threepinespress.com

© 2023 by Frieder Anders

All rights reserved. No part of this book may be reproduced in any form or by any means, electronic or mechanical, including photocopying, recording, or by any information storage and retrieval system, without permission in writing from the publisher.

9   8 7 6 5 4 3 2 1

Printed in the United States of America

Translated from the German, *Abwehrkraft: Leben mit Taiji*, by Livia Kohn

First Edition, 2023

⊗ This edition is printed on acid-free paper that meets the American National Standard Institute Z39.48 Standard. Distributed in the United States by Three Pines Press.

Cover Art: Design by Brent Christopher Wulf based on the German original. Photograph by the author. Calligraphy of *jin* 勁 (internal strength, inner power) by Wang Ning.

Library of Congress Cataloging-in-Publication Data

Names: Anders, Frieder author. | Seitz, Emanuel, 1973- author.
Title: Living with Taiji : resilience through inner power / by Frieder Anders with Emanuel Seitz.
Description: First edition. | St. Petersburg, FL : Three Pines Press, 2023. | Includes bibliographical references and index.
Identifiers: LCCN 2022055233 | ISBN 9781931483711 (paperback)
Subjects: LCSH: Tai chi.
Classification: LCC GV504 .A64 2023 | DDC 796.815/5--dc23/eng/20230109
LC record available at https://lccn.loc.gov/2022055233

Contents

List of Illustrations — iv

Preface — vii

Part One—Taiji in Action

1. What Is Taiji? — 3
2. The Internal Tradition — 11
3. Lineage Structures — 21
4. Practice, Study, Cultivate — 30
5. Sports and Games — 41
6. Weakness Wins — 56
7. Taiji and Medicine — 62
8. Breathing Types — 73
9. True Inner Power — 85
10. Testimonials of Master-Disciples — 98

Part Two—Fundamental Concepts

11. Basic Principles — 113
12. Inner Power — 126
13. The Daoist Perspective (by Emanuel Seitz) — 135

References — 152

The Authors — 154

Index — 157

List of Illustrations

Fig. 1. The Taiji Symbol. Source: Public domain.
Fig. 2. Coat of Arms of Niels Bohr. Source: Gjo; Wikimedia Commons. License CC BY-SA 3.0, 3/8/2010.
Fig. 3. The Eight Immortals. Source: Mural in temple in Hue (Vietnam). Public domain.
Fig. 4. Zheng Manqing. Source: Public domain.
Fig. 5. Master Chu, ca. 1981. Source: Public domain.
Fig. 6. Chen Weiming (left) and Yang Chengfu (right). Source: Yang 2005.
Fig. 7. Inner Power is Like a Pnedoulum Ball. Source. ©Axel Gaube.
Fig. 8. The Newtonian Pendulum. Source: Public domain.
Fig. 9. Dong Yingjie. Source: Public domain.
Fig. 10. Movements from a Peking Form. Source: Public domain.
Fig. 11. A Statue of Bruce Lee in Hong Kong. Source: Benson Kua, "Statue of Bruce Lee at the Avenue of the Stars;" Wikimedia Commons. License CC BY-SA 2.0, 7/5/2009.
Fig. 12. Yang Chengfu and Yang Shouzhong. Source: Public domain.
Fig. 13. Zhang Sanfeng. Source: Public domain.
Fig. 14. Yang Luchan, 1799–1872 Source: Public domain.
Fig. 15. Yang Jianhou, 1839–1917. Source: Public domain.
Fig. 16. Yang Chengfu, 1883–1936. Source: Public domain.
Fig. 17. Yang Shouzhong, 1910–1985. Source: Public domain.
Fig. 18. Chu King-Hung, b. 1945. Source: Public domain.
Fig. 19. Frieder Anders, b. 1944. Source: ©Axel Gaube.
Fig. 20. The Big Fish in Taiji. Source: Infobono on Pixabay.
Fig. 21. Master Chu in 1985 and in 2021. Source: Anders 2015.
Fig. 22. *The Great Learning* Classic. Source: Public domain.
Fig. 23. The Word "Heart." Source: Calligraphy by Wang Ning.
Fig. 24. Happy *Qi*. Source: ©Axel Gaube.
Fig. 25. Feet First, Then Body. Source: ©Axel Gaube.
Fig. 26. Tree, Rooted yet Relaxed. Source: Photograph by Ramaz Bluashvili, www.pexels.com.
Fig. 27. In Tripod Position beyond Earth. Source: Photograph by Cash Macanaya, www.unsplash.com.
Fig. 28. Changing Mental Status in Preparation for Action. Source: "Libet-Experiment;" Wikimedia Commons. License CC BY-SA 3.0, 6/27/2011.
Fig. 29. Round Arms. Source: ©Axel Gaube.
Fig. 30. Anatomy of the Elbow. Source:
Fig. 31. Double Helix. Source: Design by Rafeeque, www.pixabay.com.
Fig. 32. Exhaler and Inhaler. Source: ©Frieder Anders.
Fig. 33. One-legged Stand, Lunar Forward Position, and Solar Forward Position. Source: ©Frieder Anders.

Fig. 34. *Wuwei*. Source: Calligraphy by Wang Ning.
Fig. 35. Push-hands with Partner. Source: ©Axel Gaube.
Fig. 36. Pulling the Ox. Source: Photography by Cuong Art, www.pixabay.com.
Fig. 37. Best Posture for Inhalers and for Exhalers. Source: ©Frieder Anders.
Fig. 38. The Tripod Position. Source: ©Matthias Emde.
Fig. 39. Seated and Standing Qigong Practice. Source: ©Frieder Anders.
Fig. 40. Body Pillar and Gate of Life/Destiny. Source: ©Matthias Emde.
Fig. 41. Limp Hands versus Tense Hands. Source: Photographs by Daria Shevtsova, www.pexels.com; and by Francisco J. Cesar, www.pixabay.com.
Fig. 42. The Humunculus Diagram. Source: ©shumpc / Adobe Stock.
Fig. 43. Lung Meridian and Fascia Line. Source: ©Frieder Anders.
Fig. 44. Tiger Mouth. Source: ©Frieder Anders.
Fig. 45. Bent-wrist Mudra. Source: ©Frieder Anders.
Fig. 46. Stretched-wrist Mudra. Source: ©Frieder Anders.
Fig. 47. Left and Right Hands in Relation to the Brain. Source: Public domain.
Fig. 48. Gene Kelly and Fred Astaire. Source: ©Photo 12 / Alamy Stock Photo.
Fig. 49. Master Chu in 1984 and in 2022. Source: Public domain.
Fig. 50. Moshe Feldenkrais. Source: Photograph by Bob Knighton. ©International *Feldenkrais®* Federation. Used by permission.'
Fig. 51. Fritz Frautschi. Source: ©Fritz Frautschi.
Fig. 52. The Common But Wrong Posture for Deep Breathing. Source: Photograph by Iva Balk, www.pixabay.com.
Fig. 53. The Crucifixion of Christ. Source: Etching by Moritz Coschell.
Fig. 54. The Gate of Life. Source: Public domain.
Fig. 55. The Pillars of the Diaphragm. Source: Public domain.
Fig. 56. Three Elixir Fields with Gate of Life. Source: ©Jerry Alan Johnson.
Fig. 57. The Immortal Embryo Emerges. Source: Public domain.
Fig. 58. The Rune *Ing*. Source: Public domain.
Fig. 59. Two Triangles Make up the Diamond. Source: ©Frieder Anders.
Fig. 60. Head Positions of Inhalers and Exhalers. Source: Gerhards 2016, cover art.
Fig. 61. Frieder Anders, 1960. Source: ©Frieder Anders.
Fig. 62. *Qi*. Source: Public domain.
Fig. 63. Chinese Neck Support for Sleep. Source: ©Frieder Anders.

Preface

An old Japanese treatise says, "Mastery is none other than the patina that comes after years of tireless polishing." The development of true superiority in human beings is like the care of precious stones. A newly cut, freshly ground stone refracts the light harshly and sharply; only a stone that its owner has polished with dedication over many years develops a soft and profound shine, a real charisma and an independent character.

Mastery, that beyond-the-ordinary skill, requires the same ongoing care and attention. Letters, certificates, seals, and other documents cannot replace the digging, grinding, and polishing of one's own person. The dumb rock of the uncultivated self to practitioners is a raw material worth working with. In order to refine it, they grind it into shape and even after a given shape has been attained, they still continue to cultivate their skills every single day, otherwise it—like the stone—becomes dull and plain. Behind every gem, no matter how small, lies a spoil heap of the rejected.

Mastery is a word alien to the modern West. People here miss a natural sense of amazement, a reverence for the monstrous, a respect for a life that cares about nothing but getting good at a trained skill. Mastery is not a competence that makes you flexible; rather, it ties people to performing the same activity over many decades. This tie to the highest as a guiding principle is not subject to benefit calculation and contains no good answers as to wherefore and why. The expense of a fully mastered skill can never be calculated in terms of material or monetary values or anything it is intended to serve. Seen from that angle, it is both useless and meaningless.

But it is precisely from this futility of constant polishing that overarching meaning emerges: the master sees the world through a lens that he has created for himself. He has learned to see the world as it is and not as he wants it to be. His gaze has become sharper, clearer, softer, and yet untroubled. He has reached the principle of the highest: the Great Ultimate—Taiji.

This book is the product of decades of practice in personal seeing and feeling. Frieder Anders has practiced Taiji for almost fifty years, served as a teacher for over forty years, and applied its methods to nourish life for over twenty years. He was one of the first Europeans to take the Far Eastern call for championship seriously. First, he became the 6th-generation lineage holder of the Yang-family style, then he did what all disciples do who truly honor their teacher: he broke with his master, not because he lacked gratitude but because he wanted to develop Taiji further and go beyond what he had learned. Since then, he has continuously improved the traditional form with regard to the different breathing types.

In 2013, Frieder Anders began publishing regular, monthly blog posts on his website which, in revised form, form the first part of this book, entitled "Taiji in Action." Everyday observations, newspaper articles, sporting events, scientific research, and mythological material all offered an opportunity to think about the right form of breathing and the best attitude to develop with regard to body and mind. His work combines Far Eastern wisdom with cultural criticism and a teaching of the Taiji techniques. Over time, the blog entries developed into a textbook of a different kind: a reader, a manual, even an oracle, a gathering of pure blossoms on just how Taiji works best in life.

Following this, the second part of the book is entitled "Fundamental Concepts." Here Anders summarizes the key principles that underlie his teachings. Anyone who has developed an ordinary into a great skill can well imagine how difficult this is. Not everyone skilled has the ability to teach, and even fewer have can put what they have mastered into words. People often feel what is right but when asked to name this, language fails them. They can show but not explain. After all, every principle is only a hint and a pointer to the right starting point, from where each disciple must find his or her own way.

The last chapter in this part presents my contribution. Called "The Daoist Perspective," it introduces the elementary vision of ancient Daoism that forms the foundation of both Taiji and Qigong. Techniques of caring for life, they are much more than health exercises or body-building methods. Originally part of a Daoist and medical system of nourishing life, they provide easy and gentle ways of healing diseases, improving health, and enhancing vitality. Daoists see an inherent superiority, perfection, and even immortality as the true nature of human beings, and their full realization as the ultimate purpose of human life in this world. Their vision is a transcendence without God based on self-cultivation and consistent practice.

Anyone who wants to follow this path is exposed to all sorts of bad, disruptive, and harmful influences. Nothing is as common and universal as the will to prevent other people from practicing. Inner power and freedom are often confused with the constant possibility of distraction and indecisiveness. To combat this, Taiji trains the mind: from determination and softness, a supple strength of defense develops, which wins without fighting and makes life easier, leading to great resilience and strong inner power.

—Emanuel Seitz

Part One

Taiji in Action

1
What is Taiji?

The Unity of Opposites

> Whoever understands the Dao does not focus only on himself:
> he is connected to the whole world.
> —*Huainanzi*

Everyone these days knows the yin-yang symbol, in Chinese is called *Taijitu*, that is, "the symbol or chart (*tu*) of the Great (*tai*) Ultimate (*ji*)." In many Eastern wisdom books or advertisements, it is usually used to mean something like the unity of opposites or an expression of inner harmony. The symbol appears on packaging for teas, cosmetics, organic food, as well as massage offers and wellness product—all kinds of consumer goods that promise well-being and balance. It expresses the cliché of relaxation culture and reduces human life to the values of inner peace, stillness, and serenity, but does not represent the art of Taiji. Its movements are gentle and relaxed, but their prime purpose is not relaxation.

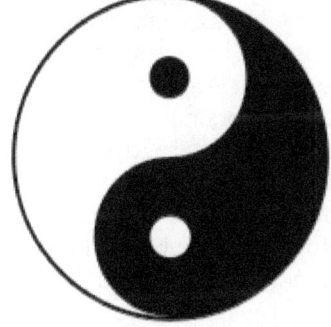

Fig. 1. The Taiji Symbol.

The meaning of the symbol also goes deeper than the cliché of inner harmony. It expresses a polarity of complementary opposites that together form one whole. The whole day consists of the period of daylight and that of darkness: they are completely different yet form one whole. Similarly, the earth contains two poles, north and south, again being completely different. There is also no inner harmony between them moreover, but the tension of the magnetic field. This tension between two complementary opposites that yet join together to form a whole is represented in the Taiji symbol.

The higher unity of opposites is called the Great Ultimate in Chinese cosmology, where it first appears in the *Yijing* (Book of Changes). It shows both the highest principle and the fundamental way of working of the cosmos. Something arises, reaches its pinnacle, then declines. Once the decline is complete, its opposite arises, and the cycle continues. Where there is a force, the must always be a counterforce. These complementary polarities, these integrative opposites, have to come to together to form the whole of anything in the world. As pure forces, they are called yin and yang. This symbol accordingly shows yin as the dark part, representing the principle of compression and condensation of force, while yang appears as the light section, indicating the principle of expansion and the release of power.

Taiji, in other words, is about much more than a mere feel-good ad to sell a wellness product to the receptive public. But enough philosophy already! Let us take a look at Taiji as a movement art and see how it works with the unity of opposites. The full name of the method is Taijiquan. The last word, *quan*, literally means "fist" and by extension "fighting" or "martial," but in its broadest sense it refers to intentional movement in a set sequence. That is, Taiji—the common abbreviation for the full term Taijiquan—always comes in specific forms, the heart of the entire system.

Some people see Taiji in the context of human movement as sport. And while it shares some of these characteristics, it is also not sport. Westerners tend to see sport as a way to control and enhance the body in a rather one-sided way. Here the body is merely as a tool toward a perfect performance, the realization of an ego that controls it, challenges it at will, and pushes it to its limits. That is, Westerners typically view the body as a machine that has to work until muscles and tendons are exhausted. Through sports training, the machine optimizes its performance, measured systematically by pedometers, heart rate monitors, training apps, or amphetamines.

Taiji is not sport in this sense, but presents a strong alternative for people who find the dominantly mechanistic approach to the body one-sided and lacking. Here the body and its movements are perceived as an integrated organism that has a life of its own. So stop using dumbbells, looking at the stopwatch, or holding on to the smartphone! You don't need to have such a level of control over your movements to do Taiji. The smooth flow of the motor processes activated during practice does not aim at increasing the performance of the body as machine, even though it may well begin to function better. Also, there is no question that the body can also be viewed as a machine in Taiji, matching the mechanics as they have been successfully studied over the past several centuries and are the subject of sciences such as biomechanics. Taiji does not contradict the findings of science—on the contrary.

However, there is a great deal more to Taiji, and the mechanics are not the only truth. In addition to the mechanical body that one has, there is also the organic body that one is. The latter eludes conscious volition because it cannot be intentionally posited and has its own independent organic life. Taiji unites the two and makes both accessible. On the one hand, it teaches how to control the body with its biomechanics; on the other, it creates space to its organic flow. In other words, practitioners train the body materially as an object of biology and at the same time energetically as the place where vital energy or *qi* flows. Thus develops the entangled unity of having and being a body.

It is like a miracle. When learning the movements, we put the processes together almost mechanically, but over time the organic flow of the movements emerges—as if of itself—guided purely by consciousness. We can let go of ourselves, release into the flow of the movements, as focused yet open attention increasingly takes over the task of controlling the body. This attention must never flag. As we practice Taiji, we must never switch off the mind even after we have learned the movements and surrendered to the feeling of flow, maybe supported by some Chinese-type background music. The mind must always be one step ahead of the movements throughout our whole life in Taiji.

The whole of Taiji is therefore both: a material body mechanism that we can control and an energetic-organic event that we can desire but not manipulate. This energetic event has a life of its own that we can only allow. We should always try to consciously perceive this life of our own and not lose ourselves in it. Instead of using the terms "material" and "energetic," one could also say that Taiji has both, a comprehensible and tangible aspect.

This brings us back to the yin-yang symbol. Because only from the synthesis of both aspects, only from their polarity does a kind of Taiji arise that really deserves the name. Neither the technical repetition of the correct movements nor the release into an indefinite soft flow allow us to reach the goal. This, moreover, does not only apply to Taiji: rather, each and every physical movement occurs between the poles of having and being a body. The ultimate and highest state appears in the integrated unity of these opposites.

Since the discoveries of modern physics, this unity of opposites is no longer the privilege of mystics.

Fig. 2 shows the coat of arms of the physicist Niels Bohr (1885-1962), which he designed for himself. It contains the Taiji symbol, because he discovered the principle of complementarity. This means that it is perfectly permissible for two observations or interpretations of a phenomenon to be valid at the same time, even though they appear logically to be mutually exclusive. In quantum mechanics, light is both a particle and a wave, showing the complementarity and ultimate oneness of the duality of wave and particle. Bohr chose the Taiji symbol for his coat of arms because the principle of complementarity appears so powerfully yin-yang thinking.

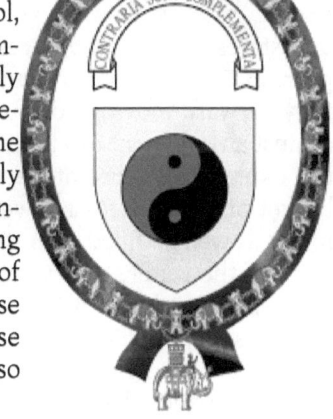

Fig. 2.   Niels Bohr's Coat of Arms.

The unity of opposites means that they complement each other and, as a result, the knowledge and implementation of complementary opposites is the highest level of being, that is, the Great Ultimate or Taiji.

The Watercourse Way

> Nothing under heaven is as soft and weak as water.
> Yet for attacking the firm and strong
> There is nothing as effectual that can replace it.
> —Daodejing 78

Many see this ancient statement of wisdom as expressing the essence of Taiji. I learned it from Karlfried Graf Dürckheim (1896-1988) who, in 1973, introduced me to Taiji at his practice center in the Black Forest, changing the course of my life. Alan Watts (1915-1973), too, influenced me greatly, notably his book, *Tao: The Watercourse Way* (1975). Both had one thing in common: they combined Western and Eastern thought to teach how to live life as if flowing "like water."

What, then, can water teach us about Taiji and thus about life? First of all, it is a metaphor for a fluid, gentle kind of movement. All Taiji should be performed softly and fluidly, like water; at the same time, it should flow incessantly like a great river. In practice, you move playfully around obstacles, dodging them with ease, yet you also strive toward a goal without wavering—just like a mighty river pushes to the sea. "Swimming in air" the Chinese call this soft form of self-assertion.

At the same time, water also symbolizes perseverance. Constant dripping wears away any stone. It has stamina, tenacity, and persistence, qualities you must develop while learning Taiji. Although soft, flowing, and persistent, water can also be very powerful. When it rises in a storm surge, it devastates towns and villages, even kills people. This great force also appears in Taiji, but it does not manifest in little extras on the edge of a peacefully forward-moving solo practice or in intense nudges when pushing against an opponent in a fight or a partner during push-hands. Pushing does not express the force of water as flow; they only have the strength of a bucket of water used as a weapon. The hard weight of the bucket, which might as well be filled with stones, is what provides the effect, not the soft force of the water. When this soft force becomes strong and devastating, waves and whirlpools arise.

As such, the inner power of Taiji can seize a person, drag them along, and carry them away. In practice, this means that inner power only unfolds when you softly play around opposing resistance. The opponent must not find anything hard, and you must not act against him. By playing along, you seduce him and lead him into a round movement, a circle—more precisely—

a spiral. The opponent can no longer escape from this spiral and is caught in a maelstrom.

How to imagine that? It is very difficult because it remains abstract as long as you have not experienced it in actual practice. Still, let me try to show it in an example. If someone grabs your wrists and holds you tight, you instinctively want to resist, using muscle strength, body weight, momentum, or contortion. If the opponent is stronger, none of this will help. What is the alternative? Certainly not surrender to the aggressor without a fight or giving up. Non-violent self-reflection may be useful, but the best is to use the way of Taiji, to become active in the manner of water.

How to act like water, then? You do so by not fighting the strong force directly, but allow the attack to happen and let it run into empty space. You play around the opponent like swirling waves of water, especially where a hard force hits. That is to say, you evade the attack by walking around the attacker and thus avoid being hit. If you cannot avoid it, you give way, just like water gives way when a swimmer enters it. Pushed out from one place, it immediately crops up in another, then reclaims the space it was expelled from and makes the swimmer's movements come to nothing.

In actual practice, this means subtle micro-movements, hardly noticeable from the outside, that render an opposing force null and void. The attacker suddenly feels no resistance and there is no longer a physical or even psychological point of attack. At the moment of impotence and confusion, you turn his energy against him, pushing him out of your space like a wave, throwing him back on himself physically and psychologically. Such are actions that follow the "watercourse way." Very much soft and weak, you retreat and yet simultaneously press the opponent with a reactive force, using current and counter-current. As a result, you force him to move, he loses his footing and soon falls.

But the goal of Taiji is not to vanquish anyone. The most adepts hope to achieve is that an attacker should lose his solid, strong, and apparently invincible form, because he is not willing or has not yet learned to follow the watercourse way and is thus bound to experience what it means that "the weak overcomes the strong."

The Quest for Immortality

> Be still, be pure; do not tire your body; do not confuse your life force, and you will last forever.
> —Zhuangzi

Both Taiji and Qigong have close ties to the Daoist quest for immortality, an endeavor that goes back several millennia and has profoundly shaped Chinese culture. As a particular practice, Taiji goes back to the mid-17th century, while Qigong began in the late 1940s as a modernized form of traditional healing exercises (*daoyin*). In both theory and practice, however, both have their origin in medical and Daoist methods of self-cultivation, such as nourishing life (*yangsheng*) for physical enhancement and nourishing the spirit (*yangshen*) for mental and spiritual advancement. Often generically called "nourishing inner nature" (*yangxing*), both serve to improve well-being, extend life expectancy, and raise the person to a higher, more cosmic, and spiritual level.

More recently, modern scientists have discovered the topic, notably phrased in terms of anti-aging or "undoing aging." For example, the German magazine *Die Zeit* has a headline, dated 4 April 2018: "Not immortal, but forever young? Aging researchers want to remedy the cell damage that comes with age."[1] In the article, Christian Honey asks whether we can soon live to be hundreds of years old and remain healthy and fit. He cites the British age researcher Aubrey de Gray as an important voice in this debate. He believes that it is likely that someone born today could live to an average of a thousand years. According to Honey, when presenting at the Undoing Aging Conference in Berlin, none actually used the word immortality, however, what else would the ultimate result be?

Modern science differs from the beliefs of traditional Chinese, who in fact worked toward the impossible and openly admitted that they desired immortality. Both medical doctors and Daoists developed potent practices for self-cultivation that served to stop aging, reverse the flow of entropy, and eventually transform life so that it never ceased. The result was a kind of superhuman figure or immortal (*xian*). Mystics in life, after transforming into pure spirit, they lived on as immortals on the isles of the blessed, on inaccessible mythic mountains, or in deep caverns in the earth.

Wolfgang Bauer summarizes their nature based on the work of the retired official and would-be alchemist Ge Hong (283-343):

> Some perfected immortals rise up into the clouds in their bodies and fly about without flapping any wings; others ride up into heaven on misty chariots harnessed with dragons. Some transform into birds or beasts and roam the blue clouds; others yet plunge deep into the rivers and seas or flutter to the tops of famous mountains.
>
> Some eat primal essences or consume immortality herbs; others mingle with people who never even become aware of their strange nature. Some hide themselves so that no one sees them; others have strange bones growing on their head and wondrous hair sprouting on their body.
>
> They all love the profound and the simple and do not dwell on the ordinary and fashionable. Such people are granted eternal life without death, but they first have put aside all human feelings and keep away from splendor and joy. (Bauer 1971, 157)

---

[1] www.zeit.de/wissen/gesundheit/2018-03/unsterblichkeit-altern-zellschaeden-alterungsprozess-therapien-sterben. Accessed 8/2/22.

Daoist images show immortals accompanied by various symbols such as cranes, pine trees, peaches, mushrooms, flowers, flutes, or gnarled staffs. Some are male, some female: with freedom from death also came liberation from any form of gender identity.

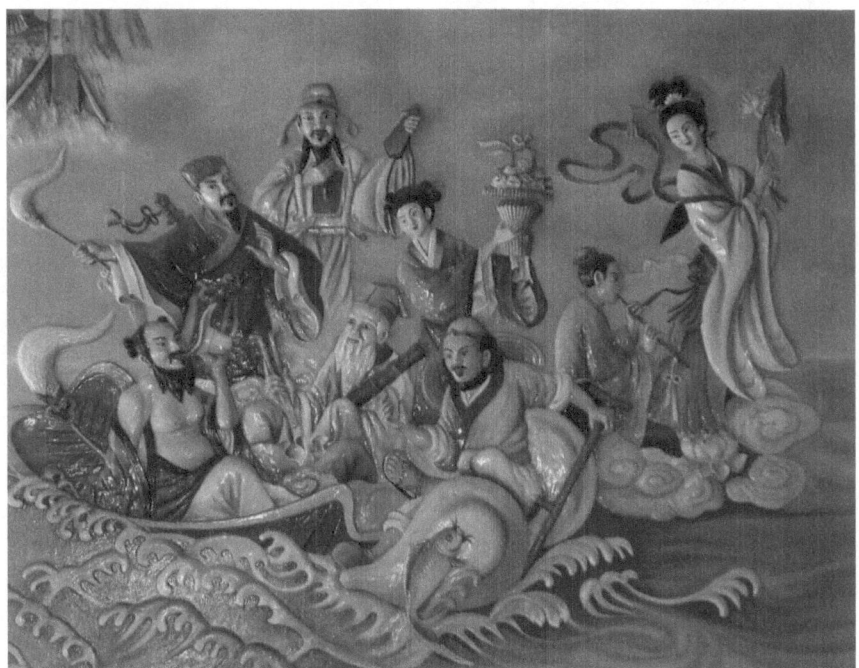

Fig. 3. The Eight Immortals.

In order to become an immortal, one had to make the body light, moving toward a purer level of energy. Methods in this context include breathing and physical exercises, fasting, dietary and sexual techniques. They all would take away the earth's heaviness during life and enhance the transformation into spirit. Ideally practitioners removed themselves from society and lived as hermits; some also practiced alchemy, searching for an elixir to conquer death. Often their concoctions, heavy on found poisonous substances such as mercury and arsenic, rather conquered life, precipitating a speedy exit into the otherwold.

Then again, there was emotional self-cultivation that aimed at "losing joy in order to gain joy." The ideal was to be free from emotions, notably the intense and powerful ones that harm the organism, reaching a state of nonaction and detachment that would offer a new level of joy and happiness, a purified serenity and internal well-being that goes beyond earthly wins and gains. In some cases, successful immortals even ascended to heaven in broad daylight; others died in appearance, vanishing from their coffins or leaving behind an object like a sword or staff instead of their corpse.

Ascetic practices have largely disappeared from Taiji and Qigong today as has the intense quest for physical immortality. What has remained, however, is the idea of gaining physical lightness through practice, notably by "rooting." A particular adaptation to gravity, this allows qi to circulate smoothly and helps to relieve aging. The lightness that is acquired through Taiji is not just an idea, but the practical experience of many who want to share it with the world every year on World Taiji and Qigong Day, since 1999 the last Saturday in April.

2

The Internal Tradition

My Personal Path

> Taiji is an internal system of the martial arts. When the movements are performed correctly and the inner principles are understood, then this is Taijiquan. If the movements are not performed correctly and the inner principles are not understood, then there is no difference from the external martial arts. Even if the movements look like Taijiquan.
> —Dong Yingjie (1897-1961), Yang-style Master
>
> Time does not transform us, it only unfolds us.
> —Max Frisch (1911-1991), Swiss novelist

After first encountering Taiji in 1973, when I stayed for a few weeks in the retreat center of Graf Dürckheim in the Black Forest, I returned to Frankfurt, then taught myself a Taiji form that was based on an American textbook by Zheng Manqing (Cheng Manching, 1902-1975). At that time, I also worked with Wolfgang Höhn, who introduced me to the Eight Brocades in the Black Forest and learned some Taiji forms from him in Frankfurt. At that time, there were no trained teachers in Germany. The form I taught myself was a simplified version of the Yang style. A friend of mine also learned it, first with me, then in New York with William Chen, a disciple of Zheng. When he came back, I renewed my training under his guidance and, in 1975, began to teach it. In 1977, I visiting William Chen in New York and I wrote the first German textbook on Taiji, which came out the following year. Two years later, I founded my own school, again the first in Germany.

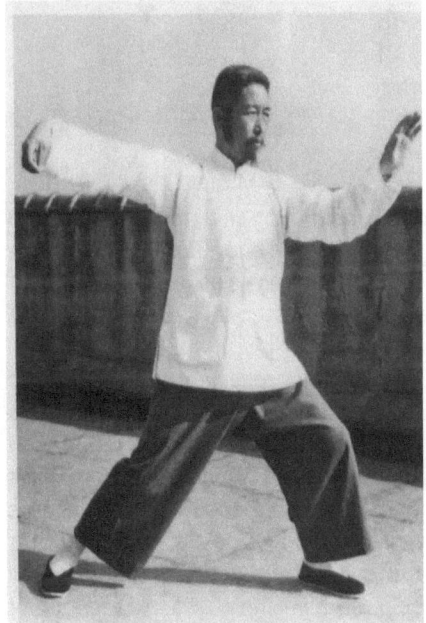

Fig. 4. Zheng Manqing.

Throughout this period, however, I was also looking for other teachers. In 1975, I contacted Master Chu King-Hung through an advertisement in London and took one week of private lessons with him. In 1978, I studied in Taipei with Master Wang Yennien (1914-2008), a representative of a different branch of the Yang style and the original teacher of Wolfgang Höhn. I went to Taipei specifically to decide which form to make the center of my focus.

As luck would have it, Chu King-Hung was there at the same time. I was walking through a park on my first day, when Wang Yennien was not teaching, and someone called out to me, "I know you!" Immediately I responded and we greeted each other joyfully. It turned out that Master Chu was visiting his family who had emigrated from southern China in 1949. He soon took me to Gan Xiaotian, a disciple of Zheng Manqing. After two weeks of working with him, I decided that he would be my primary teacher there, mainly because Master Chu had led me to him.

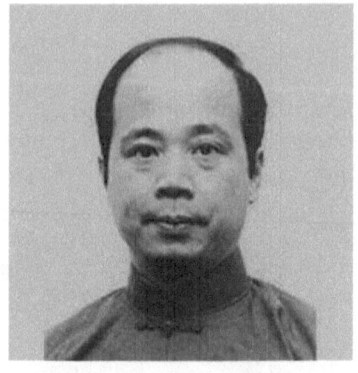

Fig. 5. Master Chu, ca. 1981.

In early 1979, I went to London to see Master Chu for a few days and began my training with him that was to last for twenty-six years. At first, I did not fully recognize his qualities in Taiji, so in the summer of 1979 I went to Taiwan again, where, in addition to lessons with Gan Xiaotian, I also attended practice with Henry Wang, another representative of Zheng Manqing's variant. However, after that, I studied exclusively with Master Chu. I told him, "Master Chu, in four days with you I have learned more than in four weeks in Taiwan!" He responded, "Four weeks? Four years, more likely!" His form soon replaced William Chen's system in my school and it is still the form I teach today, just refined with the breathing types.

In 1988, Master Chu appointed me first as a master-disciple and, in 2002, he recognized me as the first European master of his lineage of the Yang-family style. We parted ways in 2005, but I owe a great debt of gratitude to him, especially with regard to the path of internal Taiji. In return, I was happy to represent his International Tai Chi Chuan Association (ITCCA) in Germany and Switzerland and brought him many disciples and teachers who helped spread his form all over Europe. After our separation, I was free to explore the phenomenon of individual breathing types, which I had first discovered when I underwent voice training, with my students and fellow teachers and eventually came to a deeper understanding of the essence of internal Taiji.

What Makes Taiji Internal

The question now arises whether Taiji is not generally internal because it is one of the internal as opposed to the external martial arts in China and why we should differentiate between Taiji in these terms. The problem is that once you learn Taiji, whatever the style, you do not automatically gain inner power. But inner power is the touchstone for real Taiji, which Master Chu described as internal Taiji. Without inner power, Taiji is a mixture of exercise and external martial arts.

A key master in this context is Chen Weiming (1881-1958), a disciple and collaborator of Yang Chengfu (1883-1936), the great 20th-century master of the Yang family. He describes inner power as follows:

> Many people practice Taiji today, but not the real Taiji.... With true Taiji, your arm is like iron wrapped in cotton. It is very soft yet feels heavy to someone trying to lift it....
>
> When you touch the opponent, your hands are soft and light, but he cannot get rid of them. Your attack is like a bullet going straight through something (*gancui*)—without the help of "sluggish power." If pushed ten feet, he feels a little movement but no power. And he feels no pain....
>
> If you use [sluggish] force, you may be able to move it, but it is not *gancui*. When he tries to use [sluggish] power to control you or push you away, it is like trying to catch the wind or the shadows. There is emptiness everywhere. Real Taiji is really wonderful. (Chen 1928, cited in Draeger and Smith 1978)

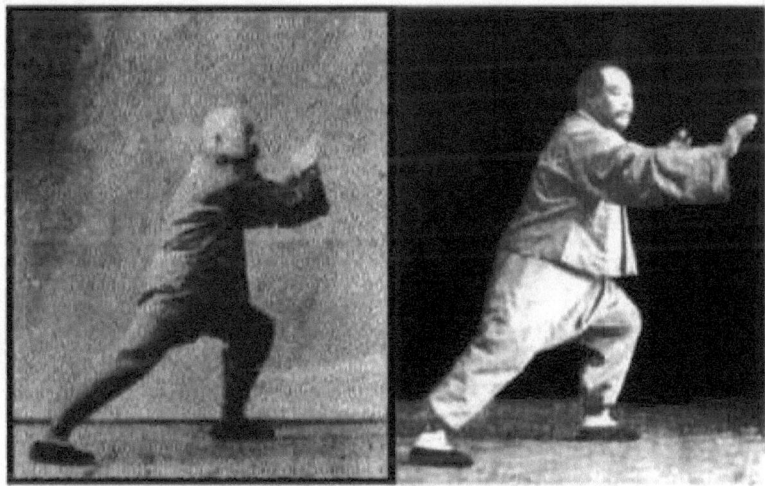

Fig. 6. Chen Weiming (left) and Yang Chengfu (right).

14 / Chapter 2

The expression used here, *gancui*, is part of the Chinese saying, "crisp and smooth" (*gancui liluo* 乾脆俐落), which means doing something straightforward and direct, appropriate to the situation. When inner power is activated, it appears soft and smooth, yet is hard to crack, as illustrated below.

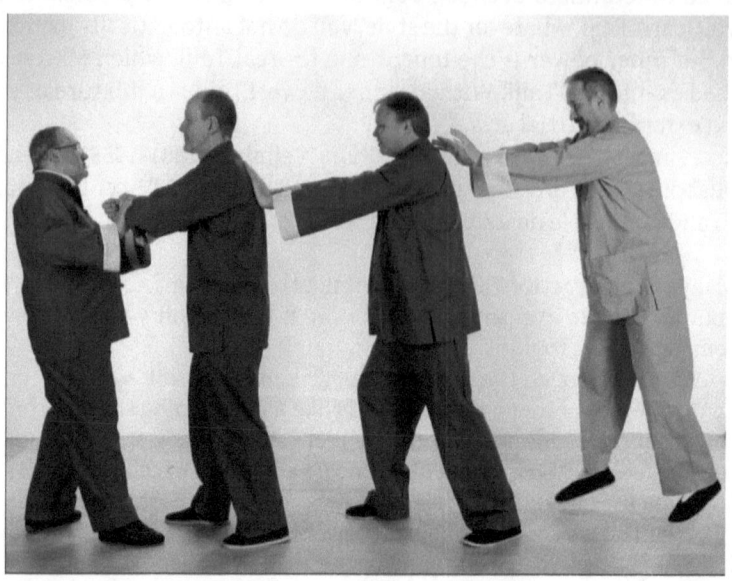

Fig. 7. Inner Power is Like a Pendulum Ball.

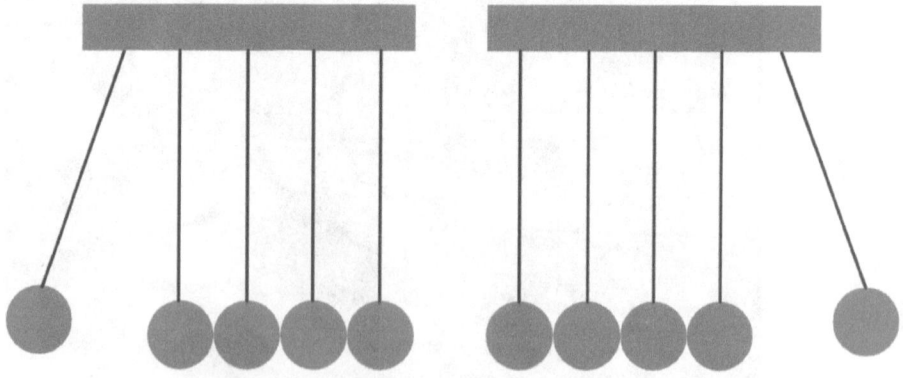

Fig. 8. The Newtonian Pendulum.

To me, Taiji is external when it only develops and applies force on the outside, an external force that invades the opponent's space and attempts to move, injure, or destroy him through intentional and voluntary muscular tension. The force finds its target in the other body, where it is supposed to explode. It is internal when the opponent is not the target of any particular movement and power comes from universal infinity and leads beyond him back into infinity. The move itself has its own infinite cycle, with destinations far beyond the opponent's body.

This marks a major difference. Through internal practice, we generate energy spirals free from intentional or voluntary muscle tension: they pull the other person in or push him away. We do not attack an opponent with the greatest tension, nor do we deprive him of space. Rather, we let him be carried along and moved away, so that he does not feel pain. When moved by pain, outward force and external Taiji are at work. But if the opponent feels a light yet strong power, the active force is inner power engaged through internal Taiji.

Many 19th-century Taiji classics say, "Even a slight deviation will lead you miles astray." This may seem daunting to begin internal Taiji, but do we really have to be that perfectionistic? Taiji is the living interplay of body, mind, and breath, and of course you have to coordinate all components in their interplay precisely, so that vitality and inner power can develop. But exercise of the body does not produce the perfection of machines. Such a claim would deprive us of being human, being alive.

All the masters I studied with mainly practiced external Taiji and thus had deviated from the right path. Some may never have started walking on it. The only exception was Chu King-Hung, who taught me true internal Taiji. Saying this, I do not want to denigrate the efforts and achievements of others. However, to me the core point of practicing Taiji is the growth of inner power, whether disciples are aware of this or not. Seekers should pay close attention when representatives of Taiji who have no inner power try to create its appearance with various tricks such as supersensory gags. Anyone who claims to be able to put out burning candles without touching them has no real inner power, but maybe secret assistants or a talent that has nothing to do with Taiji. In order to develop inner power, it is essential to work with one master who has it without bragging about it. No need to travel the world: just come to Frankfurt.

The Origins

Internal Taiji was the most famous martial art in China in the 19th and early 20th centuries. Its main hallmark was not fighting but letting any attacker bounce off by uprooting him energetically. External practice, on the other hand, was all about force and reaction speed.

There are clear distinctions between internal and external martial arts as well as between internal and external Taiji. The terms do not echo the level of martial involvement but describe the way power is grown and trained.

People tend to look for the method that suits them best, yet power is the goal of all martial arts: without power any art would be considered inferior. Their representatives—and there were about 400 different styles at the time—regularly competed and fought with each other to prove their power

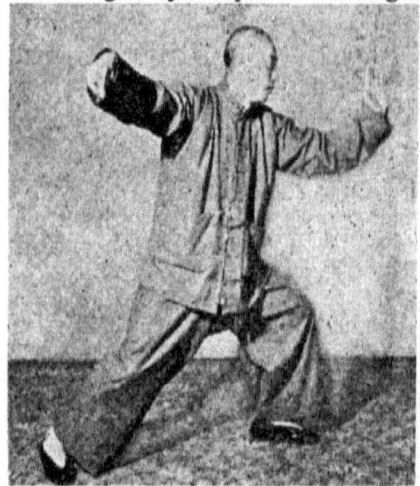

Fig. 9. Dong Yingjie.

Although Taiji was considered an internal martial art, it could also become external. Dong Yingjie (1898-1961), a 4th-generation Yang-style master, writes: "Taijiquan is an internal system: When the movements are performed correctly and the principles are understood, this is Taijiquan. If the movements are not performed correctly and the inner principles are not understood, then there is no difference from the external martial arts, even if the movements look like Taijiquan."

In the external styles of martial arts, practitioners developed arms and legs into deadly weapons, coupled with great reaction speed: the credo was "eye, fist, and foot." The limbs hardened and developed a strength of humongous proportions. In the "tiger-claw style," for example, people trained to rip pieces of bark out of trees with their bare hands. The same was done back then, often successfully, with the skin of opponents. However, the power here is merely external, mechanical force.

The development of power in an internal martial art uses mind and breathing in such a way that the body reacts like a ball hit by a hard object, that is, it rebounds. The motto of internal Taiji is *yi, qi, jin*: intention, energy, and inner power. With mental guidance, the relaxed body and internal *qi* grow the core feature called *jin*. Rather than working with involuntary muscles, one needs to develop spontaneity and empathy. It is all about the right tension in fighting: if you are too hard and tense, you lose; if you are too soft and weak, you do not get anywhere. It is quite like a kite-flying competition, using pieces of broken glass glued to resin-soaked strings. If the line is too loose, the kite cannot take off; but if the line is too tight, the opponent's line can cut it even with a small movement, and the kite is lost. Just as the cord must not be stretched taut, muscles cannot be overstretched.

Inner power comes from the right, upright posture that connects heaven and earth. It grows from the feet to the head, lengthening the physical body into a connecting line from the center of the earth to the north pole. This line becomes the central axis, the world-supporting pillar, the Great Ultimate that gave Taiji its name. From the basic mental attitude of uprightness and connection comes a superiority that goes beyond mental and physical strain, emotions and the will to win. Despite this superiority, however, Taiji as a martial art does not hurt, even if it could. The ability to survive in combat always goes hand in hand with not inflicting pain on the opponent. Otherwise, it is no longer internal Taiji, but external.

Loss and Recovery

By the end of the 18th and beginning of the 19th century, Taiji was only one martial art among others, cultivated, trained, and transmitted within clan lineages. Outsiders were generally not taught unless they showed special aptitude, motivation, and loyalty to the master. They might be adopted into the clan as disciples if they passed exams and paid substantial pledges.

The masters exchanged sons and other family members with each other to expand the learning base for initiates. Around the middle of the 19th century, families and styles became more distinct. In the course of this demarcation, Taiji emerged as a more unique martial art and styles bore the names of their founders. The Chen style is the oldest. Originally about defeating the opponent without fighting, according to Master Chu, it has today "lost its secret." Opponents lose forced by pain, in contrast to real inner power which brings them gently to the ground, "like going to bed," as Master Chu can impressively demonstrate.

After 1912, when China became a republic, the old masters lost their courtly sphere of activity, the teaching of high officials and soldiers. They looked for new students and made efforts to make the art accessible to anyone interested. To this end, Yang Chengfu, the 4th-generation lineage holder of the Yang style, unified and simplified the form without depriving it of its inner power: he just made it easier to learn. The masters traveled, taught, and exchanged ideas. As fruitful as this period was, it also brought about a leveling off. Due to their many absences, masters lost direct contact with their students and thus control of their lineages. Masters would stay on site only in brief intervals before they traveled again, leaving the bulk of the training to a one or several senior students. Despite this, the inner circles of the families were still able to cultivate and preserve the secrets of internal practice.

This changed in 1949, with the beginning of the People's Republic. The communist rulers were suspicious of anything that did not fit their dominant worldview. They considered all inner power as superstitious magic and tried to break with all old traditions or at least appropriate them in their own way. Many Taiji masters emigrated or hid their inner power and no longer demonstrated it in public.

In 1955, a new mode called the short Peking form was created. Based on the Yang style, it takes about five minutes to perform and was intended to provide the masses with a means of gaining better energy before going to work. There was no more talk of inner power. This was followed by Peking forms of 44 and 88 movements, using numbers that had no more connection with the sacred numerology of old, where numbers like 80, 81, 108, or 124 signaled a connection with the cosmos.

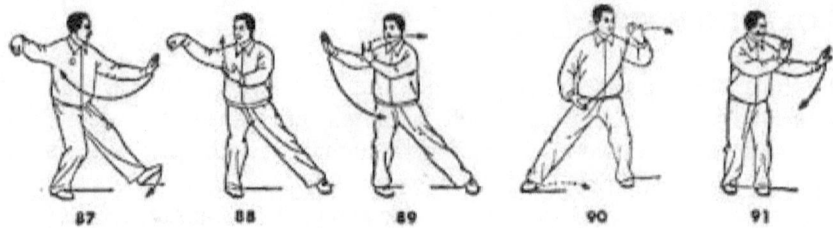

Fig. 10. Movements from a Peking Form.

In these Peking forms, moreover, movements were modified according to the findings of Western sports medicine and martial arts, *wushu*, became the name of a show troupe that traveled around the world in the 1960s, showing moves that looked as if they matched traditional martial arts, but in face were all about elegant appearance. This was the forerunner of Eastern or martial-arts videos, later exported massively into Western movie theaters.

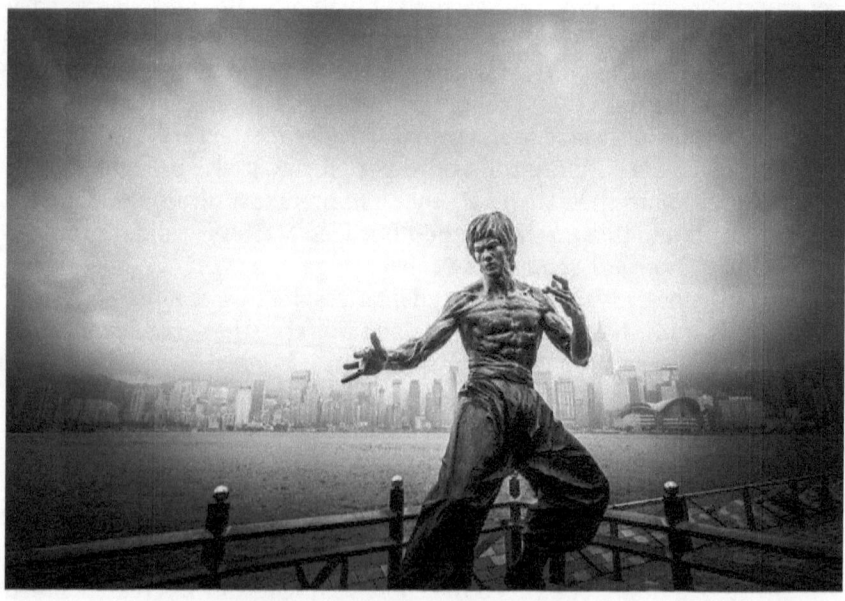

Fig. 11. A Statue of Bruce Lee in Hong Kong.

The decade of the Cultural Revolution (1966-1976) was particularly harsh. The old Taiji masters had to go into hiding or ended up in prison. Wang Peisheng (1919-2004), a Wu-style master, was incarcerated for seventeen years. Today, official sources speak of exile during this time but the one who really emigrated was Yang Chengfu's son Yang Shouzhong, a great master of inner power who fled to Hong Kong in 1949.

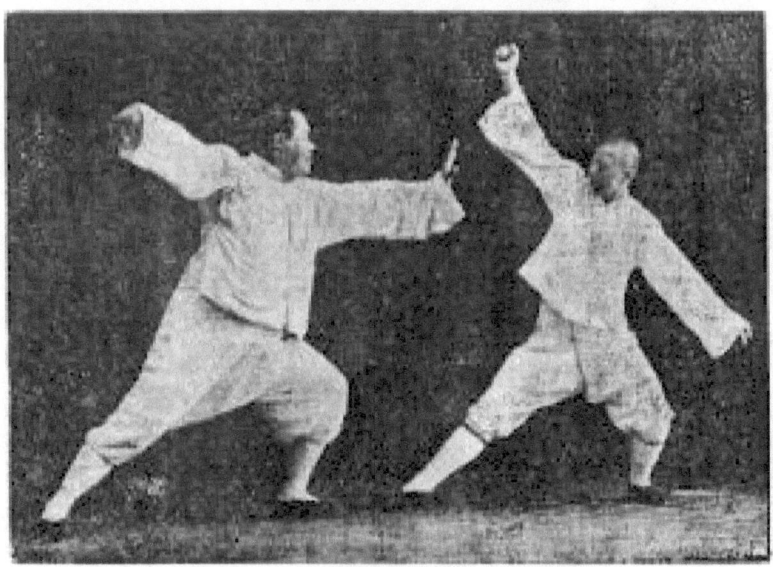

Fig. 12. Yang Chengfu and Yang Shouzhong.

Other masters who stayed in the country borrowed from the external martial arts and created a changeling: a Taiji that works with external force to be acceptable to the state. This new version was compatible with the dialectic-materialistic worldview and not endangered during the Cultural Revolution. The result was a synchronized Taiji which had lost its original internal nature.

Around this time, my first German teacher, Wolfgang Höhn, established contact with one of Yang Chengfu's nephews, Fu Zhongweng (1903-1994). He suggested that he study Taiji with his son, but unfortunately the latter only taught the official version of the People's Republic, which did not interest Höhn. The fear of openly practicing the old tradition was too great at the time. It only gradually lightened after Mao's death in 1976, leading to the Qigong boom in the 1980s and a revival of Taiji, marked among others by Fu Zhongwen teaching in Switzerland.

Masters with inner power had not completely disappeared and are still present today. Some Youtube videos show many competent practitioners, however, they work semi-underground: the state keeps them isolated and so it is difficult to get in touch with them.

In another vein, the communist government pays lip service to the tradition. In 2008, it founded the Yongquan Study Association with the official goal of preserving ancient knowledge. It focuses on historical data. For example, an article in *The New China* notes that Yang Luchan (1799-1872), nicknamed Yang Never Lose, was appointed by the imperial family in Beijing in 1850 as the emperor's chief personal guard. He also served as instructor of the imperial bodyguard and teacher of the emperor and the princes. After 1912, his son Yang Jianhou (1839-1917) taught Wang Yongquan (1904-1987), who was only seven at the time. His classmate was in turn Yang Chengfu (1883-1936), the son of Yang Jianhou. At his father's behest, Yang Chengfu took over Wang Yongquan's further education in 1917.

The journal article goes on to say that with the many different Taiji lineages, genealogy is important because it lends legitimacy to a school. Zhu Huaiyuan (1911-1999) studied with Wang Yongquan since 1934, but only became his personal disciple in 1957. Zhu was the teacher of Shi Ming (1939-2000), who called his style Ruyi Taijiquan. Starting in 1982, Siao Weijia studied with Shi Ming. In 2006, 160 former disciples of Wang Yongquan and their descendants came together for the Wang Yongquan Memorial Event in Beijing. Since then, the members of the Yongquan Study Association have met regularly.

It is questionable whether this mechanical collecting of rather technical information on the old tradition succeeds to revitalize or recover it. To date, it has not, and Taiji in mainland China has still been stripped of its essence: it is not worth the long journey to gain personal experience there.

3
Lineage Structures

Secrecy

> If people spoke only what they understand, there would soon be a great silence on earth.
> —Chinese Proverb

Chinese martial arts are like the Easter Bunny and his eggs. Tradition traces each style back to a legendary founder from mythical antiquity. The more famous the ancestor, the more important is one's own style.

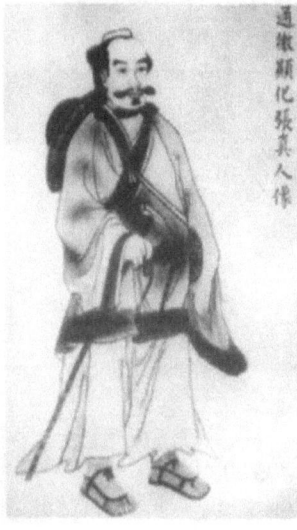

Fig. 13. Zhang Sanfeng.

Zhang Sanfeng from Mount Wudang, allegedly of the 14th century, is considered the founding father of all Taiji, and to the present day, Wudang Taiji students claim to be his direct descendants. However, it is more likely that this particular form is a reconstructed version from the late 1970s, when the People's Republic was slowly reopening. There is no trace of an old origin but, then again, people make no real attempt to ensure historical accuracy with lineage family trees.

For example, Yang Chengfu, the most famous 20th-century Yang-style master, claims that he received oral teachings from his famous grandfather, Yang Luchan, the Yang-style founder—a miracle since Yang Luchan died ten years before Yang Chengfu's birth.

Belonging to a lineage is often more important than ability. A few years ago, a legal battle raged in the US about a Taiji master named Yang who claimed descent from Yang Luchan. The Yang family resisted fiercely, claiming that someone wanted to adorn themselves with their laurels.

Yang Chengfu's three younger sons objected from China, where sons are automatically considered great masters and lineage holders. To what extent these sons were actually tutored by their father is uncertain—most likely they were taught by senior students, generally not worth mentioning. Only Yang Shouzhong (1910-1985), Chengfu's oldest son, was definitely trained by his father, reaching the rank of master. Also serving as his father's assistant and accompanying him on his travels, Shouzhong became

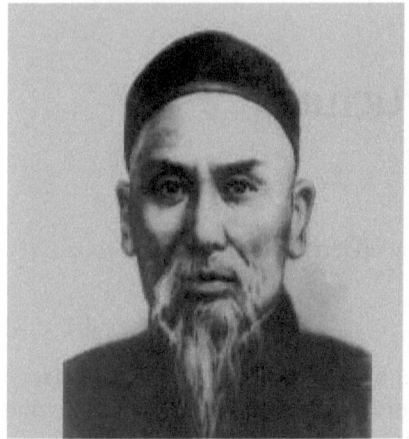
Fig. 14. Yang Luchan, 1799–1872.

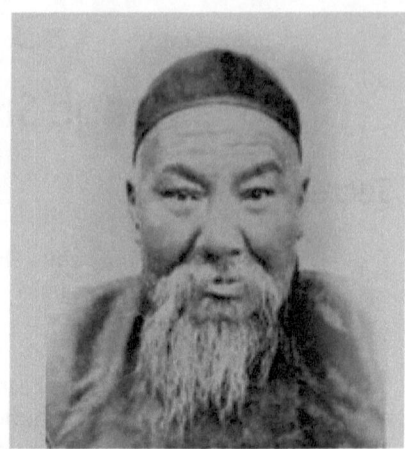
Fig. 15. Yang Jianhou, 1839–1917.

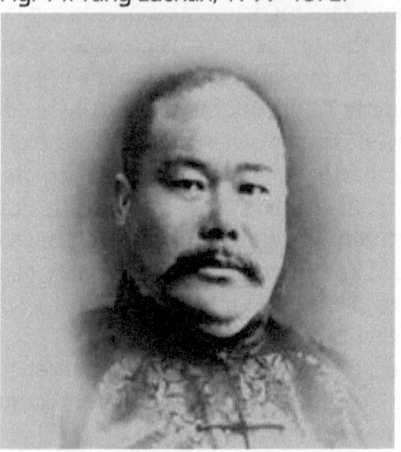
Fig. 16. Yang Chengfu, 1883–1936.

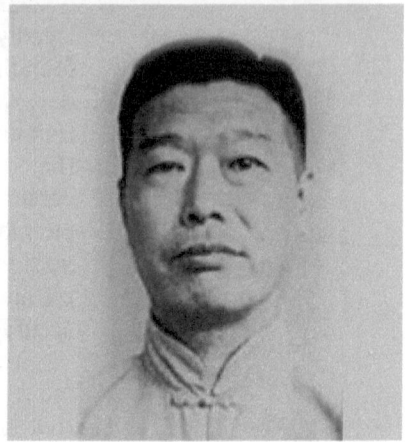
Fig. 17. Yang Shouzhong, 1910–1985.

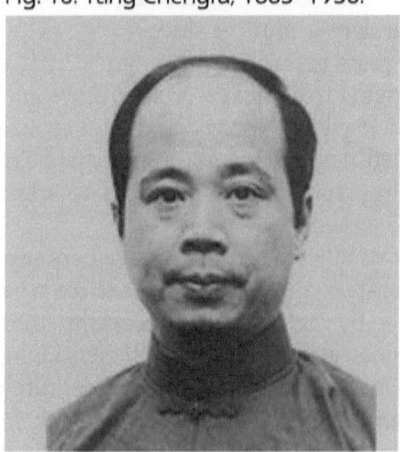
Fig. 18. Chu King-Hung, b. 1945.

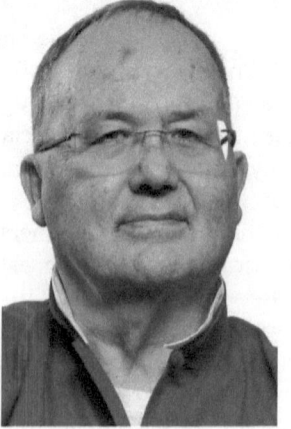
Fig. 19. Frieder Anders, b. 1944.

a leading Taiji master in his own right. But in the official Chinese version of the lineage, he is often ignored because he left China in 1949 for Hong Kong. A black sheep to the remaining family members, he did not become the official head of the family tradition, despite his abilities.

What all this shows is that being named master of a martial-arts lineage does not say anything about abilities. It simply means that the person was diligent, knew etiquette, and faithfully obeyed his teacher. Whether he also gained inner power and was a genuine master often remains unclear and is not necessary to garner respect for name and tradition.

Conversely, genuine masters often refrained from transmitting the real secrets of Taiji in order to maintain influence over their students. For example, within my own lineage (see Figs. 14-19), Chu King-Hung studied the way of inner power from Yang Shouzhong, and I studied with Master Chu. However, when I parted from him in 2005 after twenty-six years of instruction, he claimed that I had not yet learned all the secrets.

The same also happened to Helmut Schubert in Vienna, a master-disciple and branch leader of Master Chu's organization in Europe, the International Tai Chi Chuan Association. He separated from Master Chu after thirty-five years and supposedly had not yet received all esoteric aspects. Maybe Master Chu did in face keep some secrets from us but, in the meantime, I continued on the path he pointed out and further developed Taiji in the spirit of the tradition.

In China, the student is at the complete mercy of the master who determines how far he may develop. This is the dark side of the great respect for tradition as practiced in the martial arts. Attitude toward fathers and ancestors is quite different from the West: in China one has to follow the elders and practice obedience, but in the West, since Oedipus, patricide has been the prerequisite for individuation. If there were creative disciples in China who developed Taiji further and successfully established their own style, this patricide was punished: they were removed from the lineage and still are today.

And what about the Easter Bunny and his eggs? In the Chinese tradition, a student is supposed to wait all his life for the secrets of the master, like children wait for the Easter Bunny to eggs. But the mysteries unlock themselves as we explore handed-down traditions. The task then is to bring forth something creative from the traditions, to discover them and adopt them instead of dutifully imitating and sticking to the master's model. We follow in the footsteps of the masters for a while, then break out to seek what they sought.

The Old Master and the Sea

> The fishing net is there to catch fish. We want to keep the fish and forget about the net.
> —Zhuangzi

Once upon a time there was a fisherman who was a master of his art. Every time he went out to sea and threw out his net, he caught the nicest, biggest fish. And he and his family never went hungry because they could eat of it themselves and sell the leftover fish in the market.

The secret of his art lay in how he knotted his nets. He chose the right thread, used the most diverse tools, each for its purpose, and tended the net with the greatest care. Every evening, returning home with his catch, he would inspect it, spotting the smallest flaws and fixing them immediately so they would not render the net useless over time.

He passed on his art of weaving a net to his sons, but also to strangers who asked him to be instructed. If they were industrious, they soon acquired similar skills and were placed on an equal footing with sons. The table was always richly set with big fish and trade flourished.

But one day it so happened that the master did not return—the sea swallowed him up and the net with him. Now good advice was dear: a new net had to be produced quickly! But how? The skill of sons and foster sons was useless: they had helped their father when he tended the net a long time ago but never produced one by themselves.

They tried to remember and gave each other advice. But without the main net, the fish they caught got smaller and smaller and they began to suffer. Soon they started to be envious of each other and began to argue. One who had learned knotting from the master himself contradicted those who had learned the art later. The most amazing confusion arose. All the nets were different, some so badly knotted that they caught no big fish at all and only got little ones.

Because no big fish was caught for so long, over time everyone forgot what those magnificent specimens looked like. They thought that all fish were small. But because everyone vaguely remembered or at least had heard of a big fish, the controversy about the art of knotting a net flared up ever more fiercely. Everyone thought that only he possessed the true art of the master.

One showed the others the yarn, which might have been like that of the master. The next one triumphed with a tool belonging to the master, which he claimed to have acquired by personal delivery. And when still no big fish got caught, they summarily declared the small fish to be big, saying that they were the same size as those that the old master had caught. And everyone built him a monument, a stately figure complete with the old net. Then the successors continued to work with bad nets which all believed were the real thing and never realized that there were big fish to catch. But maybe there were fishermen who had secretly preserved the art of knotting a net or rediscovered it.

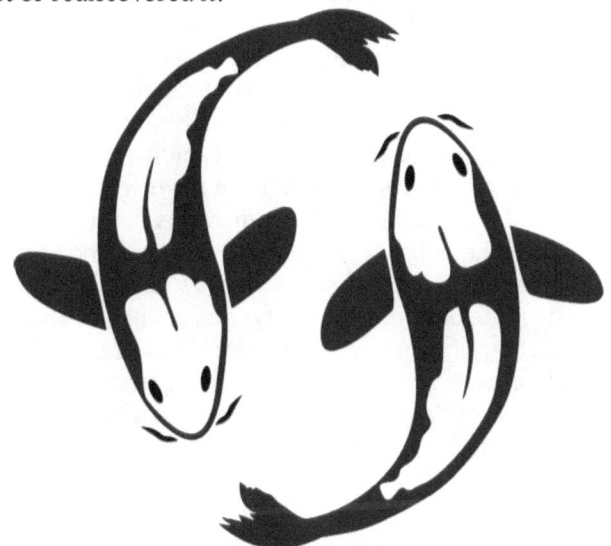

Fig. 20. The Big Fish in Taiji.

This story matches the history of Taiji, especially of Yang-style practice. Testimonials show that Yang Chengfu mastered the art of knotting the real net and landed the biggest fish: the *jin* power, the essence of internal Taiji. He had four sons. The first, Yang Shouzhong, also mastered internal Taiji, studying full-time with his father from age eight to fifteen and later serving as his assistant. Chengfu supposedly had 10,000 students, but this is where the argument about true legacy begins. Everyone who ever studied with him refers to him and claims they are his equal, just like the fishermen in the parable.

Yang Chengfu's three younger sons (by his second wife) also claim full mastery. Zhendou (1926-2020) was head of the Yang-family tradition, Zhenyi (1921-2007) taught, but Zhenguo (b. 1928) did not appear as a teacher. They knew the outer form of how the net should be, but they never really learned how it had to be knotted to catch big fish. Videos clearly show that none of them have inner power.

The oldest son, Shouzhong, on the other hand, had it. Master Chu, who studied directly with him, told me a lot about his teacher's inner power. Unfortunately, there are no pictures of him, only one video on YouTube. Chu developed his own inner power over a long time, reaching it fully only after the death of his teacher in 1985.

I had the opportunity to meet Yang Shouzhong shortly before his death and found just why Master Chu took so long to find his inner power, based on a division I make in terms of dominant breathing types. That is to say, Chu was an inhaler and thus stood upright, but Yang was an exhaler and accordingly leaned forward, matching the model of his teacher, also an exhaler. Chu's teachers could develop inner power even from this slanted posture, but for him, with his breathing type, it was impossible.

As a result, Master Chu had to change the form his teacher taught him, allowing it to be more appropriate for his breathing type. This in turn led to a situation where, even to the present day, he is reviled by Yang-style traditionalists since his form is different from the original in terms of posture and movement execution. Still, for him, this is the right way.

Now, however, he behaves just like his teachers and seems to have forgotten his former issues. He teaches all his student based on his own form developed on the basis of his body type as an inhaler and claims that his way of practicing is the only correct one, that even his own master actually practiced this way. Photos and videos clearly show the opposite.

Chu further claims Yang deliberately changed his mode for the shots so that no one would learn the only true and proper posture. However, the obvious question is: Why would he do that? Was that really necessary in his time? In fact, I am convinced, Chu has long known about breathing types, but he follows the fundamental Chinese attitude that one must not contradict a master, which would amount to patricide. On the other hand, if he did not claim to have the one and only truth, his disciples would come to doubt and contradict him. Either constitutes a major violation of the Chinese tradition and authority structure.

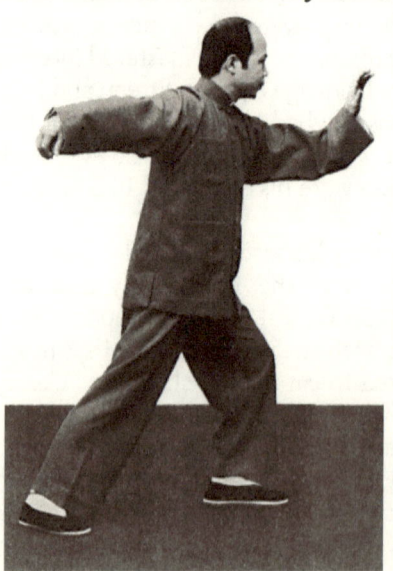 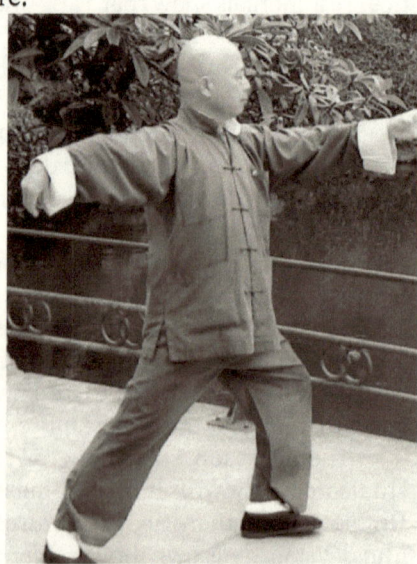

Fig. 21. Master Chu in 1985 and in 2021.

Yang Shouzhong had two other master-disciples, both exhalers who directly copied him as their model and ended up dividing his Taiji lineage in the West among themselves: Chu Gin-Soon (1932-2019) took charge of the US, while Chu King-Hung (b. 1945) taught throughout Europe. Both co-existed peacefully until Gin-Soon sent his son to France in the late 1990s to poach King-Hung's students, leading to open warfare among them.

The second master-disciple was Ip Taitak (1929–2004), who took on students relatively late in life, so that there are only two special students of disciples (*tudi*) who spread his variant of Yang-style Taiji, John Ding and Robert Boyd (aka Snake Style). Both Gin Soon and Ip Taitak had inner power as is easily visible on YouTube.[1]

Beyond all these, there is Yang Shouzhong's oldest daughter, Yang Ma Lee, who teaches in Hong Kong. For several years, she has also worked with Western disciples and founded an association with them. She claims to practice the truest Taiji ever, faithfully imitating her father's form, and insinuates that he only transmitted a third of his secrets to his leading disciples and the remaining two thirds to her alone. Again, the Easter Bunny raises its head. As long as she lives, she is the lone guardian of the treasure of tradition in the secret palace—swathed in mystery, with no presence on the internet.

While all this seems fantastic and rather absurd, I must admit that I was also like that. Thirty years ago, my teacher was the only one and the very best to me. I argued bitterly with my fellow students about how the master did it correctly, down to the smallest detail such as the exact position of his little finger. It took me quite a while to discover that the art is not about copying external movements and postures as closely as possible. Rather, it is about making them your own, giving the internal flow that the movements predicate a unique expression in your being. Students must feel and recognize what rooting feels like and get an intimate sense of what it does. After that, the rest is merely an external discussion, entirely artificial, just like this debate about who now possesses the true Taiji.

True Taiji comes about when we realize what the external net is for and what big fish Taiji wants to catch. That fish is inner power. If someone has it, they are on the right track, whether they received even a third of the mysteries through the lineage or not.

I myself gained clarity about this through experience with the breathing types. They are not part of the ancient tradition and many would reproach me that they are really irrelevant since there is no record among the old masters. Indeed, there are no records, but that is because the idea of breathing types is relatively new. Yet they applied it in practice and

---

[1] For Gin, see www.youtube.com/watch?v=WKtK-ifyasc; for Master Ip, see www.youtube.com/watch? v=eqo6jZBiVbA (accessed 8/2/22).

sensed it correctly. Images of the masters clearly testify how they moved according to their specific way of breathing.

It would all be so much better if the many sons of the fisherman Yang Chengfu (and their descendants in turn) focused on the big fish they really want to catch. I myself am just another fisherman among them who would like to teach people how to tie good nets, so that everyone can find inner power in their own way. And then, of course, once you have the fish, you can forget about the net.

Authenticity

> What you inherited from your fathers:
> Purchase it to own it.
> What is useless is a heavy burden
> It can only use what the moment creates.
> —Johann Wolfgang von Goethe (1749-1832), German poet
>
> Do not follow in the footsteps of the masters.
> Seek what they have sought!
> —Matsuo Basho (1644–1694), Japanese poet

East and West meet in these two poems. The German writer and the Japanese haiku master both demand that one should not be satisfied with a copy or imitation, but make anything a teacher or role model has created one's own, working with it so it becomes effective for oneself and in one's own time.

In Taiji circles, however, the position often prevails that only an exact copy of the model is authentic and that any new developments or individual deviations are fundamentally bad. The Chinese concept of discipleship requires that a good student follows the master with complete accuracy. Only when he has become a master himself may he adapt the art to his own needs.

This is a double-edged sword. On the one hand, teachers cannot let students stray into their own too early but they must guide them firmly to master all that the tradition has to give. Otherwise, students will just follow their own preferences, their ego, and do merely they think is right, without growing into their full potential. On the other hand, sticking to their teacher's role model for life prevents students from finding and developing their own authenticity. Key here is finding the right moment to break away from the teacher.

My own personal situation matches this conflict. It is doubtful just to what degree my way of Taiji is still authentic in relation to the forms I learned from Master Chu. I changed a great deal of his system so that, when you see him or his faithful students on video and compare their movements to what I teach, you will not find the two identical and begin to doubt whether I am in fact an authentic teacher in his lineage.

However, from my perspective, the twenty-six years of training with Master Chu have taught me what the essence of the Yang-family style is: the development of inner power. In addition, I emphasize the breathing types, which were clearly present among the old masters during its heyday from the mid-19th to the mid-20th centuries, even if they did not explicitly and systematically differentiate them

I used to call my version Old Authentic Yang Style, adapting Master Chu's expression Original Yang Style, which also appears among other students as Classic Yang Style. But what is "authentic" about it? It does not mean that everyone is doing the exact same moves. Since the early 19th century, the Yang family has brought forth numerous variants, many of which bear no resemblance to each other. It is not even clear just how the movements taught by Yang Luchan, the original founder, looked like originally.

What is authentic about the different styles and variants is the mastery of inner power. You can call on a master and his tradition as much as you want, if you do not master inner power any standing in any tradition is just smoke and mirrors. Only by growing real inner power can one pursue what the masters were seeking and not just follow in their footsteps. As George Orwell notes, the famous author of the novel *1984*: "The best teacher is one who gradually makes himself superfluous." This is because such a teacher eventually sends his students off to walk on their own feet.

4
Practice, Study, Cultivate

Living with Change

> To help all people who practice Taijiquan to long life and eternal youth. The use of Taiji for self-defense is of secondary importance.
> —Yang Luchan (1799–1872), founder of Yang-style Taiji

What is safe in my life? My job? My health? My relationships? My identity? Only one thing is certain: my death. Today, living in such a safe way seems to be harder than ever. Insecurity is part of our lives and it is growing or at least felt more severe than ever before, precipitated by rapid social change and the ubiquity of war and terrorism. A 2016 headline encapsulates the sentiment: "World Disorder Creates Anxiety."

In mind and body, we have to learn constantly to live with change, to accept it and adapt to it. One may have a strong will to hold on to an achievement or follow the erroneous belief that one must absolutely and singularly reach a goal in just the way one imagines. A mind unwilling to learn will soon sense a difference between reality and wishful thinking and perceive that difference as pain. Most of the time, this pain leads not to an openness to change but to a search for crutches—ideologies, dogmas, belief systems, justifications, and scapegoats to sustain a confused self without changing its attitude.

Daoist philosophy, on the other hand, teaches to go with the flow and adapt to change. Change is the only constant other than death, which is also understood by some religions as a transition, a transformation from one form of existence to another.

How does such acceptance of change work in practice, free from fatalistic humility that robs us of our own energy?

First of all, change in Chinese thought is not formless. The ancient classic *Yijing* defines every life situation as a moment, in which certain actions are beneficial and others are rather disadvantageous. There are sixty-four possible situations, each symbolized by a hexagram, determined through divination using coins or milfoil stalks. A hexagram consists of six lines, either two-part yin or single yang lines. The lines, moreover, themselves are changing and thus indicate a flow in the situation. For Chinese wisdom, nothing stays the same, but every situation is constantly changing because certain parts turn into their opposite.

Taiji is a way of learning how live with change in embodied practice. Each sequence of movements presents a continuous alternation of yin and yang, closely matching Chinese wisdom. Some authors, in addition, have attempted to link individual moves in Taiji to specific hexagrams in the *Yijing*, but that seems rather far-fetched to me. To me, the experience of change is most valuable, the physical turning from yin into yang and vice versa, which in Yang-family style happens about 200 times in one run. This is not just mechanical or physical matter, though. Since the spirit always leads the movements in Taiji, the practitioner also mentally practices the ability to live with change.

Over time, the practice allows adepts to survive better in their ever-changing everyday life. But this only occurs if they know about and take into account the alternation of yin and yang as a concrete event. Anyone who practices Taiji as constant gliding and floating above everything has not understood this key principle. Change or transformation from one force into another occur in separate events that do not blur into one another and become an undifferentiated flow.

The event of change is not a goal. Just how important this insight is, becomes clear in comparison to athletic performance. Here the physical process serves to achieve a specific goal—the fastest run against the clock or the greatest distance in long jump or throw. All organic possibilities are subordinated to this goal, often without regard to potential damage in health. Exhaustion and burnout are common when ongoing, dynamic change is subordinated to a goal to be achieved one day.

The linear focus on a distant goal reflects the eschatological understanding of life and world in Judeo-Christian culture. Here history is seen as having a designated end and life has a distinct goal. In ancient Chinese philosophy, on the other hand, time was understood dominantly as cyclical with only little linear progression—always circling around a center and returning to an origin. This is why at the end of the Taiji form one returns to the starting point. Change is happening constantly, moving into the form and recovering the origin.

So how should we shape our life journey? I suggest that we learn to recognize and embrace living with change. Heraclitus, a fifth-century BCE Greek philosopher, is credited with saying that "everything flows" and that no one can step into the same river twice. This thinking is very similar to Daoism, because after one dip into the river, its water changes and flows on so that the next dip takes place in a completely new river. But while the river bed—the ground you stand on—changes too, it does so much more slowly. This means, we should learn to feel how the ground supports us, even though it is surrounded by the waters of change. Then we can experience security and stability in ongoing transformation. And that is exactly what happens in Taiji: we learn to swim with the flow of time and at the same time to root ourselves on solid ground. In this sense: a peaceful journey! The end comes by itself.

Breathing Types

> I often have not eaten all day and did not sleep all night, just to think. It was no use. It is much better to learn.
> —Confucius

In 2005, when I began to study breathing types in Taiji, I came across a book that gave me important insights: *Secrets of Chinese Meditation* by Charles Luk (Lu K'uan-yü). He distinguishes between normal/natural and reverse/correct breathing. He says,

> Natural breathing, also called abdominal respiration, comprises an inhalation which reaches to and an exhalation which starts from the lower belly: when breathing in, the air enters and fills all parts of the lungs, expanding them below and pressing down the diaphragm; the chest will thus be relaxed and the belly will expand. When breathing out, the belly contracts and pushes the diaphragm up to the lungs, thus forcing out all the impure air. (1991, 171)

Reverse breathing works the opposite way: when breathing in, the abdomen contracts and the lungs fill. Upon exhalation, the abdomen relaxes and the expands below. Normal breathing is more relaxing while reverse breathing is more stimulating. Accordingly, Charles Luk recommends using one or the other mode of breathing in different situations. However, he does not go into detail about what breathing should occur when and for whom it is appropriate. He recounts his personal experience:

> When I began my practice of meditation, I found correct breathing very suitable for me and this is why I mentioned it in the first edition of this book. Since its publication, some readers wrote to me that they were unable to practice it. If it is not suitable for every meditator, I would advise my readers to practice natural breathing, which is free from all impediments. (1991, 173)

Abdominal respiration is also called diaphragmatic breathing, as opposed to thoracic or rib breathing. In abdominal breathing, according to current knowledge, the diaphragm is not pushed down by the lungs, but the other way round: the diaphragm contracts, unfolds the lungs downward, and at the same time pushes the abdominal organs down. Exhalation is described correctly: the abdominal muscles are active.

The two modes can be clearly assigned to my system of breathing types: normal breathing suits exhalers, while reverse breathing is found more among inhalers. If there had been a systematic analysis of breathing types in China, Charles Luk would probably have assigned his recommendations accordingly. But this is not the case.

The cause lies with the Confucian-influenced worship of the master. The rules of a Chinese master are rigid: "Do it just like I do, anything else is wrong." Masters would accordingly never teach a breathing type that did not match their own, preventing disciples from focusing on their own inner experiences and choose what suits them individually.

Anyone who set out to find their own path in self-cultivation or the martial arts, often the only choice was to separate from the master: either they were cast out or they broke the connection.

Another factor that has prevented systematic training according to breathing types is the immense importance of learning, another Confucian legacy. Rather than placing greater emphasis on experimentation than rote learning, learning here always trumps experimentation. The key dogma is: better learn than think (see Chua 2011).

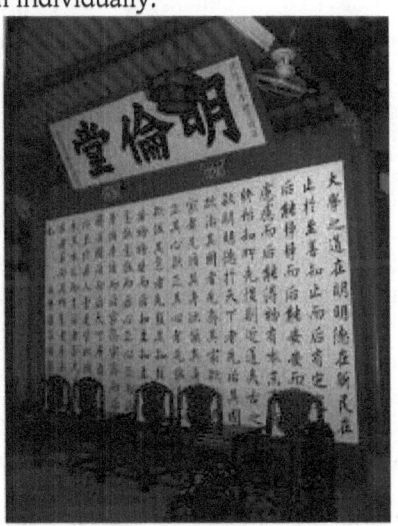

Fig. 22. *The Great Learning* Classic.

Some time ago, a young Chinese woman came to study Taiji with me. To diagnose her breathing type, I showed her the appropriate movements of the two kinds so that she could feel the difference. I very much hoped that she would have an "aha" moment, but that did not happen. She made an effort and was able to perform both types of breathing. When I asked what felt better for her, she replied that both were the same and insisted that she could learn both!

Given her cultural background, I did not blame her for being unable to relate to the feelings in her body. Under the circumstances, I could not take her on, and she will have to find her way elsewhere, with many blessings from my side. For myself, I may have failed to acquire a new student, but I gained an experience and learned something important. Internal awareness is key, even before working with Taiji.

The Self—Optimize or Cultivate?

> What we do not approach in love
> remains for us a land of death.
> —Zen saying

Self-optimization is a hot topic these days. People who want to "make something of themselves" optimize their body and themselves. A plethora of devices serves this purpose, from training, endurance, and strength machines to devices that measure heart rate, blood pressure, and everything else, thereby to optimize through feedback and focused training.

This attitude toward the body has its root in modern science. The physicist Herbert Pietschmann (b. 1936) describes this change in understanding in his Schwarzenberg Lecture of 2015, which remains unpublished to date. According to him, it goes back all the way to antiquity, because science as founded by Aristotle tolerated no inner contradiction. It was either-or, with nothing in between. The trend intensified in the Renaissance when Galileo (1554-1642) demanded for the first time: "Measure what is measurable and make measurable what is not." René Descartes (1596-1650) broke down all things into their smallest components, and Isaac Newton (1643-1727) taught to look for mechanical causes in everything. This frame of mind still shapes society today. People understand living processes as mechanisms that can be analyzed and controlled as scientists break them down into the smallest components, make their effects measurable, and find their ultimate cause.

This mechanistic mode of thinking, however, has contributed greatly to the loss of vital dynamic. Descartes divided the world and human beings into matter (*res extensa*) that can be measured and mind (*res cogitans*) that cannot be measured but does not produce any direct effects. Since then, the predominant tendency of Western thought has been to ignore the inherent dynamic of life (*res vivens*).

The Chinese concept of self-cultivation begins just where modern science leaves off, that is, with life. Its methods do not try to optimize the body by measuring and controlling it. Rather, they use, develop, and cultivate pure life energy or *qi*, focusing on a force that sits right between having and being a body.

Having a body describes the notion that the body is treated as an object, with which I can potentially do anything I want because it obeys me. I can subject it to my goals, measure it, and tweak it to work in any way I wish. I can push it around and "inject it to health" when injured or exhausted. When any of this does not work, it must be because my inner self is weak or my will does not want what my body in fact can do. This was called the "inner bastard" during World War I, a means to discipline soldiers when were at the end of their tether.

Being a body, on the other contrary, works with the body that one is. People can only perceive this body through direct experience and subjective feelings, because emotions and sensations are how it tells them what it needs and can do. Anyone actively being a body learns to listen to it and does not treat it like an object under the control of an external will. Rather, it has a will and a life of its own. Of course, such listening to the body may lead to navel-gazing and a disconnect from the outside world, but such sinking into subjective internality lacks vitality, just like the purely objective optimization of the body.

The cultivation of *qi*, on the other hand, aims precisely at the inherent dynamic of life that Pietschmann speaks of. What does that mean specifically? For example, I have had problems with a weak right ankle since I was young. I did not ruin it playing soccer, but I somehow damaged it. Western medicine could not help and as it did not work the way I wanted, I vacillated between self-pity and contempt for the part of my body resisting my will.

Both self-pity and contempt are bad attitudes. Since I wanted to impose my will on my foot and made it the object of my judgment, it remained weak and vulnerable. In other words, I did not love my foot because it was weak and so it remained weak. Contempt is driven by hate and aversion, self-pity by the desire for pleasure, an expression of the tendency to relish one's misery and even lose oneself in it. More recently, I have been able to make peace with my ankle and accept it for what it is. Since then, I no longer strain it but try to help it become more mobile with joy and friendliness. It has been getting better ever since.

Accepting the body even in its deficits is the basis of self-cultivation. It is the opposite of competitive sports, where the body is primarily an instrument that serves to achieve certain goals, an instrument injected and drugged toward greater fitness. People turning away from this often see self-cultivation as the promised land, using it to enhance their self-pity and justify their inherent laziness. Qigong and Taiji are indeed loose and effortless forms of practice. However, they are not without effort. The alternative to wrong effort is not no effort, but right effort: clearing the way for the body so that the organism can develop its capacities and flourish in its vitality. This, in turn, can be quite as strenuous as clearing land to ready it for planting.

An open heart is crucial in this process. It must be nurtured and cultivated. Mencius's statement, "Where the intention [of the heart] goes, the *qi* follows," is at the core of Taiji. But if the heart is understood in the Western sense as the seat of feelings, self-pity is not far off. It should be seen in the Chinese sense as the seat of the spirit and consciousness, that is, the mind. Never forget that we must all movements be guided by the mind, a clear mind that recognizes wrong turns and evasions.

Being like Salmon

> If you feel too old for something, you should definitely try it.
> —Picasso

During his first seminar at my Taiji school in Frankfurt in the early 1980s, Master Chu opened all our eyes. We thought that practicing Taiji meant going with the flow and taking the path of least resistance. But he made it clear that it was more a question of rowing upstream in order to realize continuous improvement and practice lifelong self-cultivation: we should go upstream like salmon and find our spawning grounds in order to fulfill our life's purpose and die.

I myself have swum upstream in my exploration of Taiji for the last forty years, after drifting for the first five. Like a salmon, I arrived at the spawning grounds after a great deal of effort, laid my eggs and should now actually die the salmon death and return to the eternal cycle of nature as food for the crayfish. That's how I felt when I turned 70, still working beyond standard retirement age yet set on an inevitable downhill course, moving toward the vast ocean.

Balderdash! What I had not considered is that salmon do not die because of their genetic programming but from stress. The biologist and brain researcher Gerald Hüther describes it as follows:[1]

> A colleague from Göttingen examined the issue and found that the salmon die from stress. They get big adrenal glands, the immune system breaks down, and then they go very quickly. He set up an experiment that I found most interesting.
>
> He helicoptered to the upper reaches of a Canadian salmon river at spawning time with a tank and took certain salmon after their mating, identified them with a red mark on their tail, and flew them to the Atlantic. After a year he checked whether he could find the salmon again. Technically, they should not be alive anymore, because salmon die after mating. But you can guess why I am telling you the story: they were back. What happened? I'll try to translate it into our language: If you're obsessed like a salmon with an idea of how things should be, then you do not see what is going on at all.
>
> These salmon race upriver, obsessed with the idea of mating, and eventually they make that idea a reality. Only then do they turn on their brain and look around to see where they ended up, where the obsession took them. They find the water extremely shallow with nothing to eat, lots of

---

[1] SWR2 Aula vom 04.12.2011 Projekt Gesundheit – wie ändere ich mein Verhalten? www.swr.de/swr2/programm/sendungen/wissen/-/id=8922982/property=download/nid=660374/1swr1co/swr2-wissen-20111204.pdf (accessed 7/4/22).

other salmon, and no chance of ever coming back. Then they have no choice but to die their brave death.

I, too, was obsessed with the idea of exploring internal Taiji to the core. This obsession led me to the source, but I never forgot the open sea from which I came, the help of the people who had accompanied me on my path or who had shown me the way. This openness of mind manifests on the persistent path to Taiji precisely because it is a path back to the origin. Professor Hüther further notes,

> I do not think medicine is there to provide euthanasia for obstinate, dying salmon but—and now I'll stop talking about salmon—medicine is there to invite, encourage, and inspire people to look for new ways, get enthusiastic about life, want to get well, trust the medical arts, and change their inner attitude. Perhaps this will allow us develop a medical system that gives many people the chance to activate their self-healing powers and get well again, and a great deal less of financial outlay.

The same holds true for Taiji. It should invite, encourage, and inspire people to look for new ways to get enthusiastic about life and activate their self-healing power, so that nobody—like the salmon—dies obstinately and obsessively an apparently inevitable death. This is especially true when they are already feeling old, as expressed in the saying of Picasso, featured at the beginning of this section.

Years ago my father gave me the book, *I Vow to Attain Eternal Youth*, for my birthday. By Johannes Kessler, Emperor Wilhelm's court chaplain, it contained sermons he held at the imperial court. I never read the thing, but the title makes a good slogan for Taiji, as is the silly phrase "forever yang," which we considered to use in ads but could not since it was trademark protected. But you have to be careful with such oaths: they may easily lead to tension and thus to an early salmon-style death due to stress.

Go Out, My Heart, and Seek Joy!

> Go out, my heart, and seek joy
> In this dear summer time
> Through the gifts of God.
> —Paul Gerhardt (1607-1676), German poet

The invitation of this beautiful song, quite well known in Germany, is highly relevant, even if summertime is often not all that pleasant but can be rather too hot. The need for joy is great. During the Covid-19 pandemic, we were under lockdown, confined to our four walls and subject to CDC rules—distance, hygiene, masking—that is, restricted in our joy in everyday life. Be it art, dance, music, sports, parties, sex, rock'n'roll, leisure, or just being with friends—everyone's heart is looking for pleasure and joy, so much more precious since we all had to do without!

What about Taiji? Can the heart bring joy and health there too – or does it just relax and calm the soul like a sedative? Master Wu Yuxiang (1812-1880) asserts, "The heart directs the *qi*." This key statement on Taiji practice means that all its movements emanate from the center of life, that is, the place of humanity.

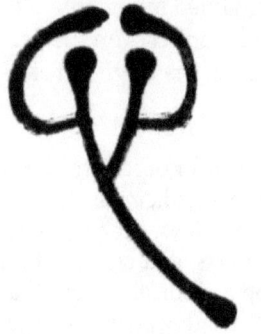

The Chinese character for "heart," *xin* 心, initially designates the physical organ and depicts its chambers. But the symbolic meaning is different. Until the late 18th century, the Chinese not only considered the heart as the seat of emotions but the center of consciousness, reason, and intelligence.

Fig. 23. The Word "Heart."

That is, "heart" in China also means what we call "mind" in the West. If this heart also directs the *qi* and has mental functions such as attention, intention, and imagination, it becomes understandable why the emotions, also centered in the heart, have no place in self-cultivation exercises. In other words, movements (as in dance) that serve to express emotions disturb the inner peace and centered quality of the meditative calm, from which the flow of *qi* should be directed. One way to get to this state is through seated meditation, described at times with the term "mind-fasting."

Calming the self through mind-fasting was a key goal of traditional Chinese medicine and the healing arts. From here, the ideal became influential in Chinese everyday life and led to a strong emphasis on moderation. "Less is more" was the motto with regard to eating and drinking as well as to material possessions, social involvement, sexual relations, and emotions. As Paul Unschuld notes, the Chinese are convinced

> that joy, sadness, anger, worry, and fear are each linked to an organ. Excessive expressions of these feelings lead to damage to the organs concerned.... Here is an example: Joy is generated in the heart. Too much joy drains the heart of its resources and weakens it. This makes the heart susceptible to heat. Those who curb their joy need not fear being attacked by heat. (2003, 86)

Unemotional calm and reasonable moderation were also part Taiji practice, understood as they were as ways to a healthy and long life.

Fast or Feed?

Besides those in favor of mind-fasting, there were also thinkers in ancient China who demanded a different way of dealing with the emotions, most importantly the hedonist Yang Zhu (ca. 440-360 BCE). He supposedly said: "A life lived to the fullest is best. A life not lived to the fullest is second. Death comes next. But the worst is a life lived under constraint" (Schleichert 1990, 80).

No writings have survived from Yang Zhu himself, but we know his teachings from the testimonies of other philosophers. He was the first to contribute the idea of "living a full life" (*quansheng*), a term that means complete life or keeping life whole, that is, enjoying life to the fullest, engaging in the emotions, and relishing all pleasures Thus he was known as a hedonist. Wolfgang Bauer notes,

> Hedonistic Daoism was about making the most of human life, which was far too short anyway, and sacrificing oneself for nothing and nobody, as quietism demanded; the hedonists turned less against society than against the planned way of life, to which a person in Confucianism was subject. (Bauer 1971, 78)

For Yang Zhu, nourishing life properly also includes a concern for joy and a serenity that does not suppress desires. He says,

> By eliminating these thoughts [of suppressing desires], one can calmly await death, whether in a day, month, year, or ten years. That's what I call nourishing life. Those who bind themselves to tyrants and do not break away from them may, in a miserable way, attain long life. But even if it lasted a hundred, a thousand, or ten thousand years, I would not call that nourishing life. (Schleichert 1990, 81)

According to Yang Zhu, anyone practicing reduction of emotions and withdrawal of the senses in mind-fasting submits only to a tyrant who blows misery into the soul or lets it dry up altogether.

Taiji is never a way to limit emotions but helps to transform them using the heart. Because emotions in themselves are not the origin of a disturbed or lost mind but an expression of the life force. The way we practice Taiji in the academy follows the guidelines of Yang Zhu. We encourage joy that comes from the heart, what Master Chu calls "happy *qi*." It is a lightness, a cheerfulness that comes from the free flow of pure life energy.

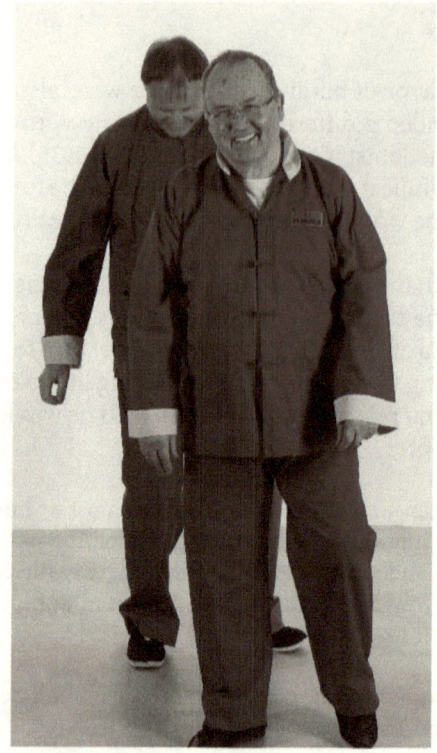

Fig. 24. Happy *Qi*.

5
Sports and Games

Playing Taiji

> People do not stop playing because they get old,
> They get old because they stop playing.
> —Oliver Wendell Holmes, Sr. (1809–1894), physician and writer

When I was in Taiwan for the first time in 1978, a man came up to me in a park ins Taipei and said, "You play Taiji very well!" Taiji in China is something one plays. I assumed that the expression "play Taiji" derives from the English expression "to play sports," which is different in German where "play" is limited to games.

In Chinese, the word is *da* 打 which means, among other things, "to hit, to make something active, to carry out." By extension, it also means "to practice" or "exercise." The character contains the radical for "hand" on the left and thus indicates something one does with the hands. This includes any kind of sport as well as board and card games. The Chinese are enthusiastic card players, and it is common to slam the cards down on the table with great force. This slamming is *da*. The term really has little in common with the general understanding of "play," the free activity of the imagination for pure pleasure.

For several years there have been Taiji schools in Germany that see their practice as a game. Their circulars and newsletters begin with "Dear Taiji Players." Unfortunately, such an understanding of the practice of Taiji is the direct result of mistranslation and thus far from authentic. Taiji remains serious business, a martial art.

When I practiced Aikido in the 1970s, I asked my teacher what he thought of Hong Kong films, which were all the rage at the time. I was interested to know if these martial arts films—pretty bloodthirsty hams— were comparable in spirit to Aikido, which also goes back to the swordsmanship of the samurai. He replied that the films lacked a serious approach to killing.

In the same way, Taiji players lack a serious engagement with combat and death. The word "play" seems to emphasize the softness of the movements and may give the impression that the movements are unfocused and free from any intention to attack. Master Chu called this way of thinking external Taiji. Although it follows some internal principles, it only uses them in an external context, preventing such players from training inner power. They tend to wait for an attack move from an opponent, then dodge it and use external power to knock him out.

With inner power, it is possible to uproot the opponent from a standing position, when both fighters are still. Dodging first and then pushing and pulling, as practiced by Taiji players, is not uprooting. Neither does it mean to knock the opponent down or off balance from a standing position with the help of holds or techniques that cause harm. Such holds block the opponent's joints, which causes pain. The practice ends up being more like Judo than Taiji.

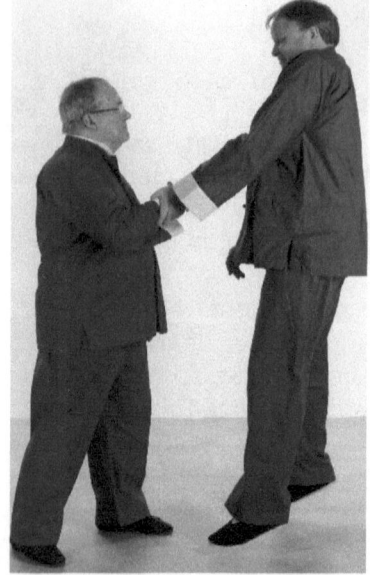

True inner power does not inflict pain. It lifts the opponent off his feet while he does not understand what is happening and how. There is no hardness to defend oneself from, but just a soft attack that just takes out his roots. The ethos of the old masters demanded that they must not want to inflict pain but still be effective in combat.

They used inner power to transform anything dark and destructive which might cause pain into something effective yet not dangerous. Taiji players who do not want to fight only want to hide destructive intentions. Truly practicing Taiji as a training in inner power transforms destructiveness into an action that is not hurtful.

Fig. 25. Feet First, Then Body

I, too, only played Taiji in my early years when I practiced Zheng Manqing's form. Zheng was a master of the classical Five Arts (painting, calligraphy, healing, poetry, and martial arts) and certainly a charismatic figure. He studied with Yang Chengfu for a number of years and emigrated to Taiwan in 1949. There he taught his own variant of the Yang style, which left out certain elements. An external Taiji developed that no longer allowed the growth of inner power. But when I started training with Master Chu, I stopped playing Taiji and began to cultivate my inner power.

Happiness and Energy

> Cheerfulness is the sun under which everything thrives.
> —Jean Paul (1763-1825), German writer

Master Chu's slogan for Taiji was simply "happy *qi*." Taiji should be performed in such a way that one feels good and can feel the energy within. This way, practitioners develop a power that can defeat another person without harming or hurting anyone. Happy *qi* means two things: subjective self-awareness and the objective ability to make a difference in the world.

How, then, can we measure happiness and energy? Is that even possible? It seems the belief is growing that it is. The trend comes from the US and is known as "quantified self." With all kinds of devices—fitness bracelets, pedometers, miCoach, and Nike+—people measure themselves consistently in order to live as healthy and happy as possible.

Trend researchers Corinna Mühlhausen and Peter Wippermann (2013) conducted a representative survey on this topic with TNS Infratest and investigated why self-tracking is becoming more and more popular. They found that health is so much more than the absence of illness and that it has lately become more synonymous with personal productivity. However, the devices not only serve to check performance but also measure just how relaxed one is.[1]

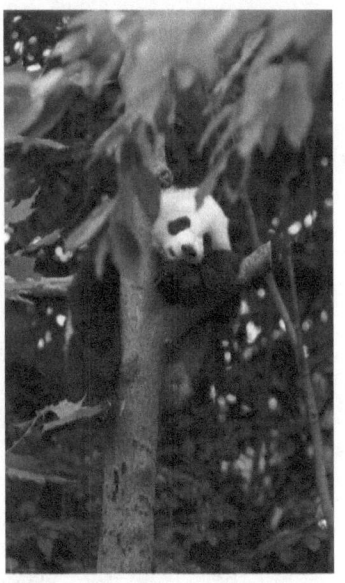

Fig.26. Tree, Rooted yet Relaxed

As harmless as that may sound, at second glance it seems frightening. Can't these people feel for themselves how relaxed they are? And why do they have to measure their relaxation right away? Are they really measuring the success of their efforts to relax?

This striving to measure everything is part of what the physicist Herbert Pietschmann calls "the mechanistic thinking of the modern age." To replace this frame of mind, he calls for a fundamental rethinking according to the principle, "distinguish but don't separate!" To him, a new holistic, integrated, or systemic thinking, such as prevails in traditional East Asia, should take the place of our limited world view.[2] He surely hits the nail on the head.

Happiness and energy are nothing in Taiji to be recorded with body measuring devices or analyzed systematically. They arise from a moving flow: this can be differentiated into individual movements but as a whole it results in an undivided movement. Happy *qi* arises from this flow.

The poet Paul Valery (1871-1945) notes, "Two things constantly threaten the world: order and disorder." For happiness to occur, just avoid

---

[1] See "Das Geschäft mit der Selbstoptimierung," by Birthe Schmidt. www.torial.com/birte.schmidt/portfolio/156043 (accessed 7/5/22).
[2] "Die Atomisierung der Gesellschaft." https://web.archive.org/web/20201203133558/; https://vorarlberg.orf.at/v2/radio/stories/2509849/(accesssed 8/1/ 22)

these two, being too rigid and ordered as well as too loose and chaotic. An order that is too rigid arises when distinctions become so strong that they separate what is connected originally; disorder comes about when differences dissolve. In Taiji, such disorder means that one indulges in an alleged flow of energy in such a way that the movements are no longer carried out properly. At the same time, however, the form must not mechanically disintegrate into its individual parts. The alternation of yin and yang creates differences but does not separate. Thus, happiness and energy are created as a whole in a state of happy *qi*.

The Taiji Pulse

> Feel the pulse of your own heart.
> Peace on the inside, peace on the outside.
> Learning to breathe again, that's it.
> —Christian Morgenstern (1871-1914), German writer

Finally! Vacation time! Finally get out of everyday life and switch off, replace the hustle and bustle with doing nothing, stretch out on all fours—*il dolce far niente*! What more could you wish for than this Italian ideal, from the country where both Europeans and Americans love to go on vacation? Doing nothing, nothing at all: for many, this is the ideal vacation, a way of true relaxation after being busy all year round by work and other commitments.

Western culture is based on the model of the tireless doer who works without stopping. Ideally, they should not need to rest at all! They organize their life according to precise goals, be they material goods, lifestyle patterns, or idealistic visions. These extend even into the afterlife: if you do not end up in hell, you will find ultimate peace on the isles of the blessed. Rest itself can become such a goal that the restless worker constantly struggles to achieve purposeful relaxation. Sleeping pills, massages, well-ness spas, or vacationing away—how far can it go?

But there is another way and that involves Taiji. Doing Taiji, one relaxes completely, but rather than being far away, one is at home; rather than lying down, one stands and moves. Between each movement there is a tiny pause when all is at rest. The two are inseparable and form a unity of doing and being. Taiji pulses with both rest and energy.

What does that mean? If you look at people practicing Taiji on YouTube, you can see that they move slowly and fluidly, in a completely relaxed way but without visible resting points. The movements flow uninterruptedly, like a great river. Yes, the whole form flows without break, yet there are frequent pauses when the movement briefly rests and the energy sinks to the bottom. In these moments, the movement culminates in a specific pose. Yet, while this happens, the mental movement keeps on going and must not be allowed to stop, as Yang Chengfu notes.

Thus, Taiji unfolds its effect and keeps on moving in a pulsating rhythm that strengthens and shapes the organism. The body itself is a pulsating structure that is rhythmically set in motion by the flow of blood and breath. It is not controlled by a ghost that makes it run like a machine.

Pulsating means that a movement ebbs and flows at regular intervals. In between is always a pause, between in-breath and out-breath or between the contraction and expansion of the heart. Without pauses there is no rhythm, but only continuous movement. Taiji movement is meant to flow, but it flows with clear waves. As the waves roll onto the beach, the movement pulses from one posture to another.

Taiji without pauses, even if done slowly, is not really relaxation but rushing in slow motion. If the biological pulse is not observed, the movement cannot have a revitalizing effect and leads to a current that ultimately makes you sluggish. More than that, this false flow in movement is ineffective and cannot be used in combat. Movements matching the pulse, on the other hand, have an effect even if carried out quickly.

The saying goes Taiji postures arose from different modes of standing meditation. The form combined these from stillness into movement in such a way that the flow of energy was not interrupted. This idea is helpful because it prevents the sequence of movements in Taiji from becoming a flow without contours. The ocean teaches us that all movement is rhythm—as should the movements be in Taiji.

For me, the road to discovering this pulsating nature was long, rocky, and winding. My first step was working with the yin-yang form. In 1985, I wrote:

> Taiji comes from stillness, hence the beginning of the form is yin. This yin phase turns into yang, then yang turns back into yin, and so it flows through the whole form, until you finally return to the exit yin.
>
> In the yin-yang form, the [initial] raising and lowering of the arms is experienced differently. The attention is no longer in the external process, but gives the movement a goal. As soon as one begins to raise the arms, one already aims at their high point, that is, shoulder height (extreme yang); when they begin to fall again, the consciousness is already at the place where this movement ends (extreme yin).
>
> The spirit's lead over the body increases, as it were, but must not lose connection. The tortoise crawling from object to object—the mind that gradually grasped the movements while learning the form—gradually changes into the eagle that surveys the distances it wants to cover from the air: the mind recognizes the form and structure of the movements. Consciousness expands, and will and determination develop, but remain connected to their base, the earth. (Anders 2015)

Keep this in mind when you go on vacation: movement and rest form a pulsating unit.

The Game of the Gods

> Soccer is the ballet of the masses.
> —Dmitri Shostakovich (1906–1975), Russian composer and arbiter

In 1999, a feature film was shot in Bhutan entitled "Game of the Gods." It shows how, when the Buddha discovered soccer, an entertaining marriage of sports and spirituality developed. As a self-confessed soccer fan, I would like to ask: Just how would early Taiji masters have played soccer?

First of all, with spirit and focused intention. In the martial arts, intention (*yi*) serves to foresee or anticipate movements. This kind of foresight is also essential in soccer, both for one's own game and to guess the opponent's moves. Intention aligns movements with a goal, whether it's a pass to a teammate or a shot at goal. Thanks to foresighted intention, a unity of body and mind is created in the movement, which at the same time relieves the mind because it is no longer lost in the small detail of individual steps. This is as true in soccer as it is in life. Alignment with goals can create a perspective that allows obstacles and resistance to be avoided before one ever has to grapple with them.

Internal Taiji teaches not to fight the power of one's partner or opponent, but to direct one's focus to a goal that lies beyond. You basically ignore the opponent's strength and attack. Exactly the same thing happens in a top-level soccer game, when a pass suddenly opens up space in a man-to-man fight. The flash of inspiration transcends the grim match with the opponent, eliminates confrontation, and gives the game a new twist from a higher perspective.

During the 2016 European soccer championship, Stefan Reinartz, a former professional soccer player, named this ability to have a higher perspective as a criterion for assessing the strength of a team. Neither matches won nor successful passes have any real significance. On the contrary, really strong teams make brilliant passes as often as possible. This new method of evaluating the performance of soccer players is called "packing." It is about an inner, spiritual dimension of soccer, about the ability to look ahead. How many opponents has a soccer player outplayed with his passes? That is the crucial question.[3]

Yi, the far-sighted, intentional mind, is responsible for those brilliant passes that make a stadium's audience erupt. The overview ensures superior sovereignty. One achieves this sovereignty if one is constantly vigilant and can therefore react immediately as soon as the opponent shows a gap. A Taiji

---

[3] Stefan Reinartz, "Eine packende Idee." www.bayer04.de/de-de/news/bayer04/stefan-reinartz-eine-packende-idee (accessed 8/3/22).

classic describes this: "Outwardly you are like an eagle circling over a pursued rabbit and about to swoop down inwardly you are like a cat stalking a mouse." This is just how the ancient Taiji masters would play soccer.

There are more similarities between soccer and Taiji, such as footwork. Also, in both disciplines the unauthorized use of arm strength is taboo—soccer rules forbid it, while in Taiji the impulse comes from the feet, continues through legs and hips, and ends in the arms. What moves from the arms is only their participation in a holistic use of the body.

Above all, however, Taiji and soccer are brothers in spirit because both use potential spirit guidance. With both, the opponent is leveraged without feeling pain—in Taiji by uprooting, in soccer by overplaying without a match. But who understands both? Who knows about Taiji and soccer? In the end I enjoy a European championship alone in front of my TV, but who knows? Maybe there is still someone who combines both.

Beyond Limits

> When the wise man points to the moon,
> The idiot only sees the fingers.
> —Chinese Proverb

Established limits are a big deal. In this context not so much political or social, but personal. On the one hand, reports are increasing of people falling ill and unable to work because they have reached their limits, that is, they have maxed out their ability to perform. On the other hand, many strive to go beyond their limits so they can face seemingly insurmountable challenges with courage and grow above themselves.

"Faster, higher, farther!" This Olympic motto coined by Baron de Coubertin today applies not only to competitive sports but all different areas of life, some quite extreme. An example disgust tests at Jungle Camp, when limits of taste are explored and overcome. The pattern is always the same: boundaries are there to be crossed. If you succeed, you reap glory; if you fail, you face disgrace or disease.

The sociologist Norbert Elias uses the term *homo clausus*, man imprisoned, for this pattern in his work *Über den Prozess der Zivilisation* (1939; Engl: 1982). What he means is that people keep trying to escape from prisons they have made for themselves. Especially since the 17th century, in an ongoing process of civilization, they have learned to control their emotions, with the result that they feel limited and imprisoned.

In addition, since René Descartes, they have believed that the inner life of every human being is a world of its own. He argued that the mind was completely separate from the body, which means that, if you try to go beyond your limits, you are trying to break through the physical constraints of your body since the mind is free to do whatever it wants. The contemporary thinker Michael Hauskeller summarizes it aptly:

> In the outer world, we assume, things are manifest in space, but in the inner world of the soul or consciousness, neatly separated from them, there are ideas, thoughts, feelings. We do not believe that they can be found outside in space, not even in our body, since it is only a thing in space. Rather, they inside ourselves, in a place that is not a place because it cannot be spatially localized. This is a spiritual domain, an intangible soul place where we somehow seem to be. From this non-place, we then look out into the world, as if from a room that has windows, but which we cannot leave, prison and refuge in one. (2004)

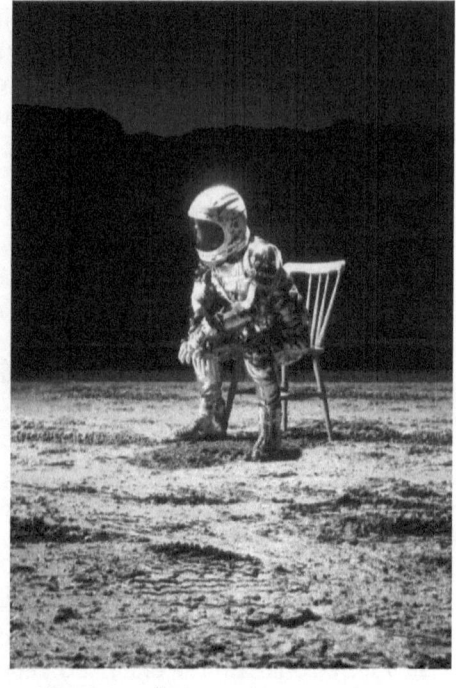

Fig. 27. In Tripod Position beyond Earth.

Attempting to push the limits of the body's capabilities is doomed to failure. As long as we cling to the idea that the will can command the body, we remain unable to break out of prison. And it is like in a real prison: we can keep fit there with sit-ups and push-ups, but we remain locked in as before.

Internal Taiji deals with the own body differently. There is no *homo clausus* who wants to break out of the body. Although mind and body are perceived separately, the mind does not command the body but guides it. There is a unity of mind and body that is nonetheless hierarchical.

A finger pointing at the moon concerns the moon and not the finger. This well-known simile illustrates the ways mind and body can interact. If you look at the finger, the mind only reaches to its end, but if you look at the moon, it goes 380,000 km beyond the limits of the body. The body becomes part of the cosmos. In this sense, the mind in Taiji should point far beyond the body. If it were to get stuck in the body, the movement would remain unrelated to the outside. If the finger—and the mind with it—really points to the moon, the *qi* flows through mental and spiritual guidance into infinity. With this extension of mind and spirit, inner power emerges.

A practical test proves again and again the effectiveness of this mentally guided energy. If the attention remains on the finger, the outstretched arm can easily be bent by another person with muscle strength. However, when the mind expands into space while the body holds the gesture, the arm can only be flexed with much brute force, if at all.

This simple test shows the Taiji way of how to go beyond the limits of the body and physical force. People practicing Western sports cannot keep up with that. The reason is simple: they do not know the moon and treat the body merely as an anatomical machine that the mind cannot influence. The strength of this body is external force, limited by anatomical capacity. The inner power of Taiji, on the other hand, is limitless because it grows beyond one's own body with the mind.

Readiness Potential

> In broad outline, the main steps of our life, we act not so much from clear knowledge of what is right as from an inner impulse.
> —Arthur Schopenhauer (1788-1860), German philosopher

There is a christmassy question relevant in love, gift-giving, and Taiji: Where does my impulse to do anything originate? Which comes first: action, will, or readiness?

To illustrate what I mean, let me recount an incident from my mid-twenties. I was living in New York at the time, working with an improv theater group. During rehearsals we practiced finding the decisive impulse for a movement or an action. It should come spontaneously and automatically initiate the task the mind was envisioning.

This is a difficult exercise, because we are used to making conscious decisions with our will before taking action rather than simply waiting for an impulse. I was supposed to become a tree in one of these improvisations and rise from a lying position as if growing out of the ground. Any attempts to will this growth and somehow do it consciously felt wrong and unsatisfying. The right momentum was missing.

Exhausted, I finally gave up, and then it suddenly happened. Something grabbed me and carried me forward into an upright position, with outstretched arms, singing loudly. I was fascinated by how the tree within me suddenly made me grow, without me doing anything. It was crucial that, despite all the fascination, I did not lose myself in this state. I experienced everything with a keen awareness and was able to reproduce what I found on stage. I call this state knowing ecstasy.

There is, moreover, a scientific explanation. In 1965, the neuroscientists Lüder Deecke and Hans Helmut Kornhuber discovered the so-called readiness potential, the unconscious impulse I experienced first-hand in New York. Measured electrophysiologically, it occurs just prior to voluntary movement in certain areas of the cerebral cortex when the body prepares for action. It precedes not only action but also the will to action. The physiologist Benjamin Libet built on this in 1979 with his series of experiments known as the "Libet experiments" (see Libet 1985).

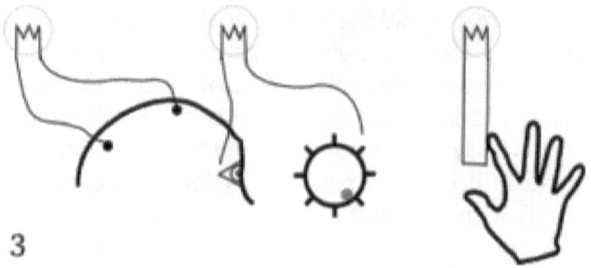

Fig. 28. Changing Mental Status in Preparation for Action.

This activation of the readiness potential is also important in Taiji. The conscious will does not go far when we try to uproot our opponent in partner practice or check inner power in tests, since it works only with the application of external force, movements of pushing and squeezing that have nothing to do with internal Taiji. The consciously managed force is directed and carried out by the ego, without the body having activated its readiness potential.

For a movement with inner power, on the other hand, one must be able to separate the impulse to move from its execution. The readiness potential comes from focusing on the task of moving someone, but being willing to act does not mean that the action must actually take place. There is still the possibility that the conscious will vetoes the realization of that willingness in a movement. However, when the movement is performed, it follows the momentum built up during the readying process. It only releases the tension has built up as readiness potential and does no more. This creates inner power and no external force or muscle strength is applied.

You can feel the readiness potential. It does not require muscular tension, where the will prepares the body for action. The more original readiness beyond muscle power arises through the mind, in the sequence *yi-qi-jin* (intention, energy, power): "Intention leads, *qi* follows, power arises."

In love and gift-giving, too, inner power arises from readiness potential. This does not mean showering the loved one with gifts and tokens of affection, which would be a manifestation of external strength, the power of money. Here, too, the will has the possibility of a veto and had better wait for the correct impulse to act.

A gift that comes from an inner impulse keeps distance and shows respect. It arises from a deep appreciation that does not believe one has to give just because the calendar demands it. In China they say: "If you are in doubt whether to give or not, better don't." Is not this omission the better proof of love and firm sincerity?

Elbow Freedom

> The head is round so that thinking can change direction.
> —Francis Picabia (1879-1953), French writer and painter

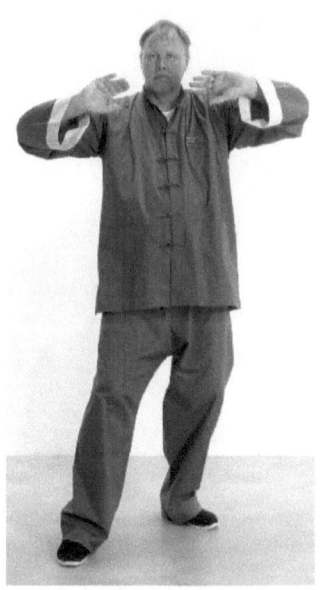

Fig. 29. Round Arms

In Taiji, the head is round and so is the body. *Qi* changes direction in its flow, and the body moves in spirals. Every movement is rounded, and even in a straight line, on the shortest route to a goal, the limbs rotate. This does not happen spontaneously or naturally—unfortunately!

Adepts have to change their understanding of movement in space: a movement that is usually flat or linear and takes place on a two-dimensional plane must become round and three-dimensional, progressing through spirals. This kind of movement grows inner power.

The elbow is key in the process. When lifting an elbow to perform a spiral movement, we merge its three constitutive joints—hinge, ball-and-socket, and radioulnar—into synchrony.

More specifically, the hinge (ulnohumeral) joint makes stretching (extension) and bending (flexion) of the forearm possible; it works both horizontally and vertically. This movement can generate great power and is used, for example, when we strike a large gong or chop wood. Any use of force where we want to move an object in a straight line uses this flexion-extension mechanism.

The ball-and-socket (radiohumeral) joint allows the forearm to rotate so that the ulna and radius rotate around each other. The radioulnar joint allows the hand to rotate internally (pronation) or externally (supination). We use this joint constantly: when we unlock a door, open a screw cap, or hold a glass to our mouth. The spiral movements in Taiji arise from the interaction of all three.

In many kinds of sports, practitioners use a combination of extending and rotating the forearm. The optimal shot in golf or tennis, for example, is always spiral. This is more efficient than flexion and extension alone, which require only external force. Because of the round movement the ball flies on a curve and can hit the target.

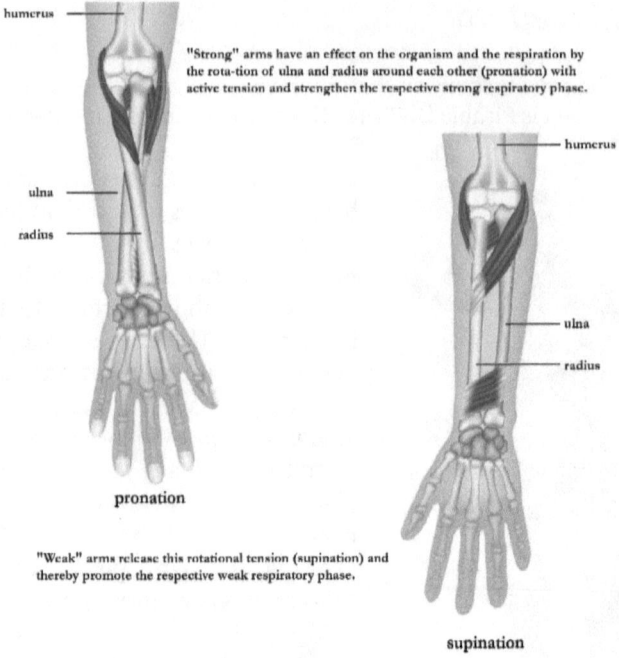

"Strong" arms have an effect on the organism and the respiration by the rota-tion of ulna and radius around each other (pronation) with active tension and strengthen the respective strong respiratory phase.

"Weak" arms release this rotational tension (supination) and thereby promote the respective weak respiratory phase.

Fig. 30. Anatomy of the Elbow

In Taiji, we use this spiral to attack the opponent with inner power, that is, we uproot him. This does not happen through a mechanical force released when we push or pull, which only uses the hinge joint of the elbow but not its ball. The elbow remains rigid and the muscles tense. Conversely, when inner power is applied, the forearm rotates on itself. The elbows remain relaxed, and flexion or extension occur from the ball-and-socket joint. In other words, the elbows are the center of a circular shape that is drawn in space with the forearms. The shoulders and shoulder blades remain in place and do not move. This is how the arm spiral is created: the arm rotates around itself.

In the mind, too, inner power does not act by mechanically countering an attack. On the contrary, the arm spiral is only effective when performed as if the opponent were not there. He or she is not fought with the help of the will, but taken in a round movement or sucked into a spiral. He gets caught in it unless he lets go. Paradoxically, the looser the twist the greater power it develops, much greater than any mechanical muscle work. It is like a gentle hug that disarms completely.

In my experience, the ability to use the three elbow joints to create a spiral is the key feature of internal Taiji. It is hard to find in videos, but has to be taught in person. Thus, at the academy, we work very hard on this paradox of gaining great strength through loose elbows.

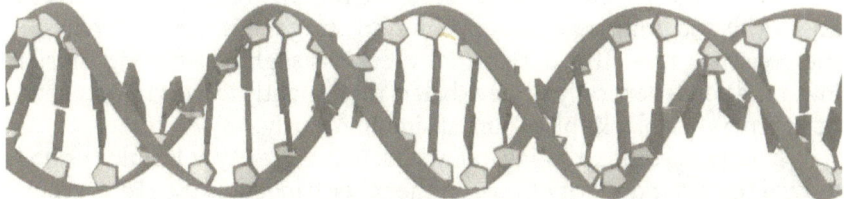

Fig. 31. Double Helix.

Especially when loose, there is a lot of strength in the elbow that can be used to great advantage. Applying it only as a straight hinge with lots of force can knock someone out but is rather clumsy in terms of elbow skills. Applying it as a ball-and-socket joint, on the other hand, opens up a great force, matching the power of original creation in nature. Be it the double DNA helix in the cell nucleus or the cosmic twirls of space, the spiral is everywhere in nature as a manifestation of inner power.

Grow into the Sky

> My art of living is: head in the clouds, feet firmly on the ground.
> —Reinhold Messner (b. 1944), South Tyrolean mountaineer

"Trees do not grow into the sky" is a widely popular saying. It suggests that one should not reach too high or serves to comfort someone whose high-flying plans have failed, that is, it is a guide toward modesty, humility, or even resignation.

But the saying is not entirely true. While trees do not grow all the way into the clouds since they are not designed to reach that far, the yet always move in that direction. Rooted in the deep, dark earth, they aim high, always moving toward the light. Doing so, they connect heaven and earth. Some trees grow bolt upright, others turn and twist like pines on the ocean exposed to many storms. But no matter how straight or bent they are, they always remain firmly rooted and grow upright as they push toward the sky.

Rooting, often also called grounding, and uprightness are key terms in Taiji. Both belong together: the upright length that reaches upward toward heaven comes from being rooted and grounded in the earth on which one stands. In the very first lesson, when I ask beginners to stand up straight, almost always the same thing happens: they stretch and their breastbone lifts, the neck extends, the spine straightens, and the shoulder blades move back. Rarely does anyone think of their feet and straighten from there, but in fact nobody can stand upright in a stable manner unless they first establish a firm footing on the ground and become aware of how gravity is holding them there.

Awareness of gravity is the first step to rooting. To do this, we bend the knees a bit and bring head and torso into an upright position. Depending on the breathing type, this upright posture looks slightly different: inhalers lower the pelvis vertically while exhalers tilt it slightly forward. Rooting and uprightness, then, take place almost simultaneously.

In physical terms, rooting follows the pull of gravity as it sinks the body toward the ground. Uprightness, on the other hand, uses the rising ground reaction force, which is responsible for the fact that we can walk upright. In internal Taiji, we make sure that only these two forces are at work, minimally disturbed by intentional muscle movements. The most natural way to achieve standing up straight, therefore, is not to stretch and tense but, on the contrary, release all tension and allow the body to fall upright with gravity.

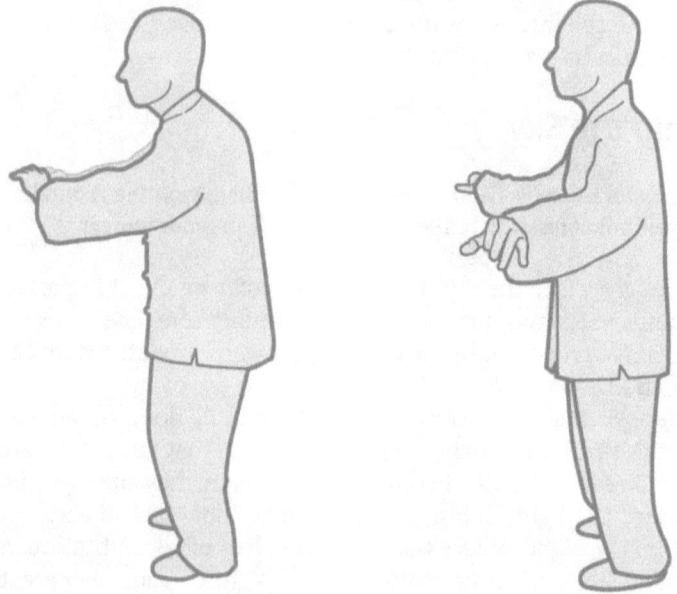

Fig. 32. Exhaler and Inhaler.

Rooted uprightness is relatively easy to achieve when the weight is evenly distributed on both legs. We practice this way of standing in Qigong. In Taiji, however, the weight shifts from one leg to the other, just as in walking. Finding the balance of gravity and ground reaction force on one leg is much more difficult here and takes longer practice. Adepts of the Yang style call this twofold engagement of the forces the balancing of heaven and earth.

Practitioners of other Taiji styles, too, claim to work with rooting and uprightness. But they tend to make the same mistake over and over: as they move, their body's center of gravity does not shift, so it keeps on resting on two legs instead of one. If one extends a line perpendicularly from the body's center to the ground, it will end up somewhere between the feet instead of one foot only. This kind of stance fails to have its axis clearly on one leg and thus can never be really rooted. In this apparent rooting, people also flex their knees, which lowers the body's center of gravity but does not lead to proper rooting. At the same time, it straightens the body from the ground reaction force. If one does it correctly, there is a single body axis at all times and in all positions.

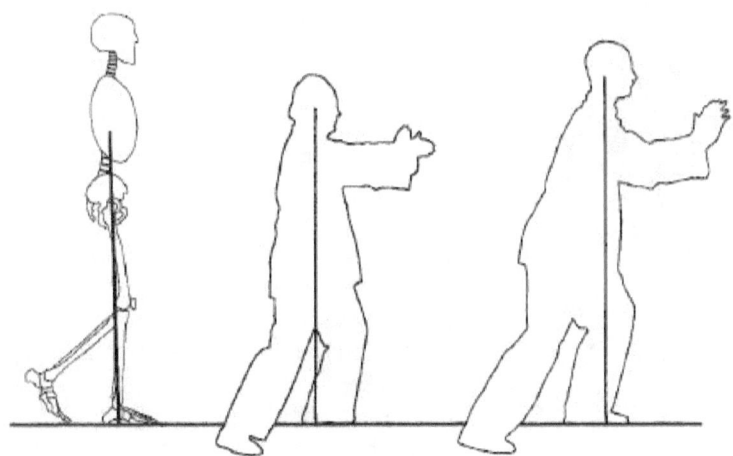

Fig. 33. One-legged Stand, Lunar Forward Position, and Solar Forward Position.

This fundamental body axis is also retained when shifting one's weight during practice. Never should the weight be evenly distributed on both legs at the end of any given movement. This is because such a weight distribution could no longer afford a clear body axis, creating several main lines instead.

Only by continuously working with a strong axis can one achieve inner power in the upright position and not stand straight woodenly like a pole. The Taiji stance means to be rooting alive and powerful in the ground; it grows upright firmly and in a stable manner, reaching well into the sky—alive like a tree not an inanimate pole.

6
Weakness Wins

Nonaction

> If you stretch a string too tight, it will break.
> If you tighten it too weakly, you cannot play it.
> —Buddha

The phrase act by not acting or nonaction (*wuwei* 無為) pervades the entire practice of Taiji. It does not mean sitting back and doing nothing but indicates an activity undertaken with highest vigilance that unfolds after a moment of pause. It is the opposite of spontaneous or reflex action.

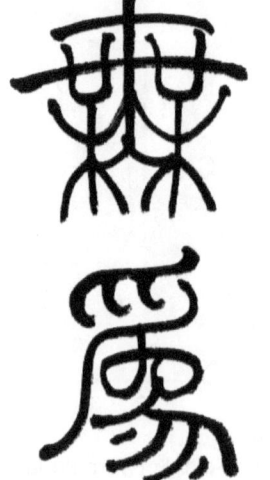

Fig. 34. *Wuwei.*

The meditation teacher Sven Joachim Haack, in a lecture at the Taiji Academy entitled "Not Acting, But Letting Go Is the Way," explained it as follows. If practitioners have a meditative experience which shows them that they have made progress on their path, they must never hold on to it and/or seek or have it again because that would keep them from moving forward.

Practicing Taiji means to look for the unity of acting and not acting. During partner exercises or push-hands, we learn to suppress the reflex to fend off the opponent, so we stand and hold back, initially not acting at all in face of an attack but letting it happen. If we allow the opponent's movement to get close and give it space, we can redirect it and turn it against him without brute force or major effort.

Instead of muscular force, we use inner power. How much this inner power affects the opponent depends on his original effort and is not part of the execution.

Inner power does nothing but reverse his external force while allowing it to continue. It is acting and not acting at the same time. It voids the unobstructed push of the other's force without fighting it with will and intention. Taiji teaches never to react directly, immediately, or without reflection. Those who can control and restrain this impulse gain a great superiority which protects them infinitely better than aggressive posturing. A counter-reaction guided by the mind has the inner power to disarm the opponent.

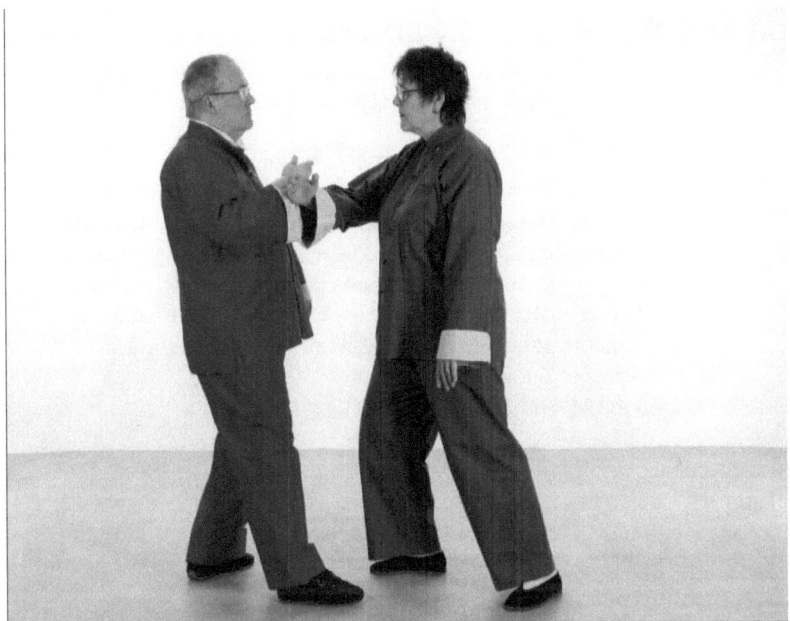

Fig. 35. Push-hands with Partner.

This reversal, when the opponent's force turns against him, happens in a fraction of a second. It takes his breath away and causes him to lose his balance, being completely uprooted. The practitioner, on the other hand, experiences this rise of inner power as liberating and exhilarating.

Nonaction, therefore, does not mean to be a passive recipient or radical pacifist who shies away from any fight. Taiji does not make you a better person in the moral sense of being noble, helpful, and good, but one can learn to refrain from action and thereby transform aggressive tendencies. If you do something against an attack but do not follow the spontaneous reflex of hitting back, you can defend yourself without hurting the other person. If the opponent hurts himself because he does and wants too much, you have not done anything yourself.

Soft and Weak, Friendly and Kind

> Kindness is a language, which the deaf can hear and the blind can see.
> —Mark Twain (1835-1910), American writer

> You cannot teach people friendliness with harshness, no matter how sparingly harshness is used.... Trying to teach people kindness through measures of harshness is the same as the proverbial war to abolish all wars. Hardness encourages more hardness; it never encourages kindness.... Certainly it is the essential ethical message of Daoism.
> —Raymond M. Smullyan (2000, 122)

Another basic principle of Taiji is to meet harshness with friendliness. This reflects its Daoist underpinning, because, as the *Daodejing* says, "the soft overcomes the hard" (ch. 36). But what does it mean? Should we really always dodge and let every attack come to nothing? Were the ancient Taiji masters really forgiving when they let opponents bounce off?

Do not confuse softness or friendliness with self-denial or meekness. Taiji does not serve the cowardly acceptance of defeat or any attitude that runs away from everything. On the contrary, true Taiji means self-assertion. During push-hands, you only give in until the opponent has maneuvered himself into an unstable position. After that, it hardly takes any strength to make him stumble and end up in a weak position. Eventually you can push him to surrender, but only after your gentle softness has allowed the attack to a certain point.

It would be wrong to understand softness to mean that we should suppress every impulse to defend ourselves. This impulse is part of our inherent vitality and instinctual self-preservation. When we give up on this, it will find another outlet and possibly turn into hate and aggression, which manifests in the hard external martial arts, whose adepts let off steam by punching a bag or fighting with force.

Taiji finds a softer outlet for this inner pressure. Potential aggression turns into inner power that triumphs over the opponent without hurting him. It keeps the opponent at a distance as it claims its own space. If he tries to get too close, he is uprooted and will harm himself. Throughout Taiji triumphs with softness and friendliness, entirely free from anger.

Anger arises when I suppress aggression and cannot find an outlet for it. It is blind and has no aim, with a tendency to get more intense when I get hurt. As holy wrath, anger is directed against any perceived cause and wants to remove or revenge perceived injustices that make me feel impotent. Unlike this, Taiji makes it possible to claim space and win in a friendly manner.

Another source for the same idea is the slogan "winning without battle," which expresses the ideal of warfare in Sunzi's strategy treatise *The Art of War* (Cleary 1988) as well as the main way of achieving victory in Taiji.

How this can be applied in everyday political life was evident in 2014 in the Bavarian town of Wunsiedel. Every year the neo-Nazis would hold parade to commemorate Rudolf Hess (1894-1987), the second-in command after Hitler. Resident deeply resented this but instead of fighting the parade with a counter-demonstration, that is, repaying like with like, they founded a non-profit charity initiative called Right Against Right (www.rechts-gegen-rechts.de). Their principle was simple: for every meter that a neo-Nazi walked through their city, sponsors donated ten Euros to the Exit Program that supported anyone who would turn his or her back on the right-wing extremist scene.

In this way, a march intended to glorify fascism became a charity that supported the opposite. Of course, the marchers only found out about their generous action against themselves after they had embarked on their way. Residents distributed bananas marked with the words: "Soon to be ripe! Part of My Feast [as opposed to My Fight] for the final sprint!" Posters lined the route with the inscription: "Fast as greyhounds, tough as leather, generous as never before!" In the end, they even gave each participant a certificate for successfully completing the charity run.

Right Against Right did not fight the Nazis, but did exactly the opposite with its strategy. They remained friendly and used the energy of the opponents against themselves. Their wit and cunning created a situation where every move the right-wingers made also worked against them at the same time: the fascists had failed and been used by their opponents.

I do not know if this win based on Taiji principles persuaded some neo-Nazis to leave the scene, but it drove the group to hold their memorial march under cover of darkness.

Nose Rings

Nose rings in traditional cultures are tools to pull water buffaloes, making them go in certain directions. Common both in East and West, they are ubiquitous in China, Vietnam, Korea, and Japan as well as bred in Italy, Romania, and Bulgaria, where they not only plow but also provide milk and cheese, notably real mozzarella. Since 2014, the animal is also bred in in the Vogelsberg area of central Germany, descending from an Italian line.

The water buffalo's nose ring is a prime example of the application of inner power. As the saying, "Easily deflect the force of a thousand pounds with the use of four ounces," indicates one cannot move the animal or an attacker with sheer physical force. Nor can he just rely on speed, such as when an old man defeats a cluster of opponents? A simple nose ring that only weighs about four ounces allows any child to control a beast many times bigger, stronger, and heavier. The child does not need his own strength for this because the nose is the ox's weak point. Although the animal is no longer in pain because callus has formed over the wound, it reacts sensitively to any pull applied.

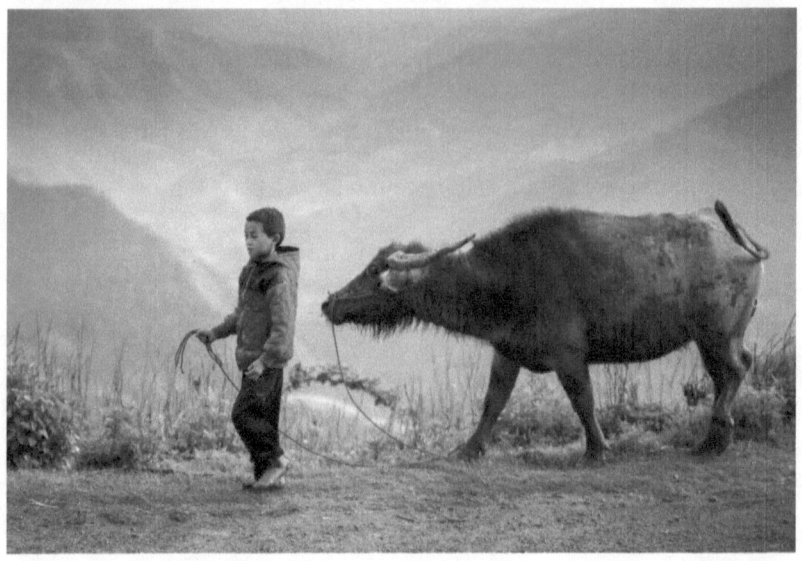

Fig. 36. Pulling the Ox.

In push-hands, adepts similarly look for their opponent's weak point to defeat a thousand pounds with four ounces. This requires a special sensitivity so one can feel when an opponent show a weakness. In fact, once you find that point, you do not need much more than a hundred grams of force to throw the person off balance. Unique to the martial arts, this uprooting does not inflict pain.

Finding the weak point without hurting anyone is different from intentionally poking a sore spot repeatedly to the point of pain. You leave the pitch as a winner, but victory is strategically unwise. Because the injured will most likely want revenge, either on you or by attacking an innocent third who he can defeat easily. From humiliation and annihilation, violence can escalate to immense proportions. Victory in Taiji, on the other hand, shows the opponent the limits he has exceeded with his aggressive attack. He is put in his place and neutralized. It is a soft win.

It takes years of practice to be able to find an opponent's weak point and put in a nose ring so that he is easy to guide. It is a long way of self-cultivation and transformation, redirecting aggressive energy and turning it into inner power. The French philosopher and sinologist François Jullien describes the strategy:

> A Chinese general makes no conjectures, elaborates no arguments, constructs nothing. He set up no hypotheses, makes no attempt to calculate what is probable. On the contrary, all his skill lies in the earliest possible detection of the slightest tendencies that may develop...
>
> The whole of military strategy, when confronting an enemy, could even be summed up by the following double maneuver: never present the slightest crack to the enemy so that he can never get a hold on you and will be bound to slide about with no means of penetrating your facade; at the same time, be on the watch the development on his side of the slightest crack, which, progressively widening into a breach, will eventually make it possible to attack him without risk. (Jullien 2004, 68-70; 1999, 121-23)

This strategy, therefore, requires a keen sense and delicate tools, the installation of a nose ring and the art to use it skillfully. Then winning comes about softly and without struggle.

7
Taiji and Medicine

Fibromyalgia

> Supple like a child, healthy like a lumberjack, serene like a sage—through Taiji
> —Chinese wisdom

Fibromyalgia syndrome (FMS), literally "fiber-muscle pain," is a widespread chronic disorder in middle-aged people. Its most common symptoms include pain in the neck, back, chest, arms, and legs, difficulty sleeping, and a general tendency to fatigue. Mentally, patients suffer from lack of drive, forgetfulness, and low productivity.

As noted by the *Ärzteblatt*, "in a study of fibromyalgia syndrome, Taiji" was found "more effective than physiotherapy."[1] It works and is recommended even by Western physicians, whose standard therapy otherwise is physiotherapy, that is, light endurance training. This serves to improve the fitness of the cardiovascular system and frees patients from their passive, immobile lifestyle. Taiji has a different approach in that, rather than raising heart rate and blood pressure, it provides a gentle and slow transformation of the body.

Another study also shows that patients were happier with this gentle way, having to work out only twice a week, and improved more rapidly than those undergoing fitness training. Randomized trials that met the strict criteria of Western medicine divided 226 patients into two groups, one practicing Taiji in a variation of the Yang style, the other working out by practicing aerobics. Doing more aerobics had no further effect on relieving FMS, while practicing Taiji created some genuine relief.[2]

While these studies provide further evidence that Taiji is effective in a clinical sense, the fact that it works is not new. A record of previous studies appears in Klaus Moegling's *Tai Chi im Test der Wissenschaft* (2009); more recent summaries of current research are found on the Taiji Academy website.[3] Backed by all this information, we can recommend Taiji with a clear conscience: it helps and there is evidence of it.

---

[1] www.aerzteblatt.de/nachrichten/92043/Tai-Chi-in-Studie-bei-Fibromyalgiesyndrom-effektiver-als-Physiotherapie (accessed 8/3/22).
[2] "Effects of Taiji Versus Aerobic Exercise for Fibromyalgia." www.bmj.com/content/360/bmj.k851 (accessed 8/3/22).
[3] www.taijiakademie.de/files/sgqt_info-dokument_qigong_taijiquan.pdf (accessed 7/7/22).

Modes of Sitting

> You can stand by your point of view, but you should not sit on it.
> Erich Kästner (1899-1974), German writer

Day after day we get bad news about death and various threatening situations. In addition to war, terror, and environmental catastrophes, even television is labeled a threat, as already documented by Neil Postman in his *We Amuse Ourselves to Death* (1988). On September 19, 2016, the magazine *Focus* upped the ante even further: not only television, but even mere sitting down kills: "More harmful than smoking: one hour of sitting costs twenty-two minutes of life."[4] The former soccer pro Philipp Lahm echoes this when he says, "Sitting is the new smoking" (2022).

The first to make this claim was James Levine who studied obesity at Arizona State University. His conclusion was: "We are sitting ourselves to death." According to him, a sedentary lifestyle is more dangerous than smoking, kills more people than HIV, and bears a higher risk than skydiving. Sitting for just two hours at a time increases risk of heart disease, diabetes, metabolic syndrome, cancer, back and neck pain, and other orthopedic problems. Not even a health-conscious lifestyle helps. "Even if you eat healthily and exercise regularly for an hour a day, but spend most or all of the rest of your waking hours sedentary, it diminishes or negates the positive effects of your fitness efforts."[5]

Oh, dear! We knew that constant sitting like a couch potato is not healthy. Nor are the potato chips we eat on the couch as couch potatoes. In addition, it has been clear for a while that sitting a lot in an office has a negative impact on health. But are we seriously doomed? Does neither exercise nor diet help if all we do is sit? One way out might be to learn how to do it properly.

This is an issue for ergonomics, a science developed to optimize working conditions to meet physical requirements, so that people do not become ill through work. It recommends a certain way of sitting, but it is rather stiff, reminiscent of disciplined sitting at school, like little toy soldiers. This is because ergonomics tends to focus on the physical body as a mechanical system and does not take into account energies that flow through it. Tight posture in any form blocks energy flow: people pull inward and tense their muscle, but do not in fact sit properly.

---

[4] www.focus.de/gesundheit/experten/sitzen-ist-noch-schaedlicher-als-rauchen-eine-stunde-sitzen-kostet-uns-22-minuten-unseres-lebens_id_5943184.html (accessed 7/7/22).
[5] https://connect.mayoclinic.org/blog/living-with-mild-cognitive-impairment-mci/newsfeed-post/repost-sitting-is-the-new-smoking/

Vibrant, energized sitting is different. It is a posture free from stress and without tension that allows *qi* and breath to flow freely. It affords freedom and pleasure, because it attunes to the body, understands it, and treats it with kindness. Proper sitting is relaxed and matches the breathing type. Specialists in breath studies recommend the following sitting postures:

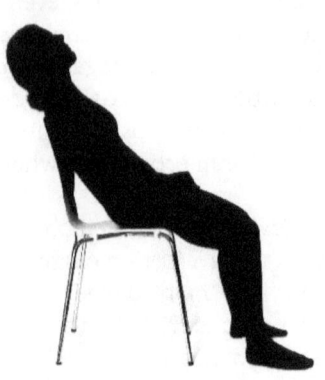 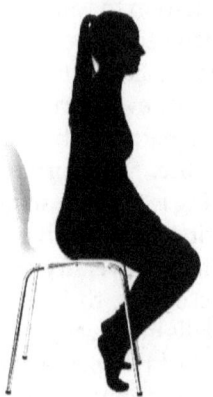

Fig. 37. Best Posture for Inhalers   and for Exhalers

Both these modes are unusual in comparison to the ergonomically recommended posture. There is no more "Head up, chest forward!" Instead, exhalers sit slightly bent forward and even pull their legs under the chair. There are no straight lines or right angles, but the posture is healthier and energetically correct. One can stay in it over long periods without getting tired. Just try it!

Another arguments word against scaremongers like James Levine is that Zen and other Buddhist monks spend much of their lives sitting down but many of them live to ripe old age or get even older than the average person. Anyone who learns to sit vibrantly, according to their breathing type and without cramping, will not sit themselves to death.

Optimal Breathing

> The weak overcomes the strong,
> The soft overcomes the hard:
> None under heaven does not know
> And none is able to match it.
> —*Daodejing* 78

What is the best posture for breathing? In an upright position as recommended by masters of calisthenics, with chest out and belly in? Probably not. While a sign of strength and role model for athletes and bodybuilders, this posture is not suitable for therapeutic purposes when a person is struggling to breathe. If there is shortness of breath, whether due to illness or as a result of excessive physical exertion, the body becomes weak. The posture it assumes naturally does not match the Western ideal of physical strength, but appears weak and passive.

Those breathing hard tend to adopt the so-called tripod position, which in German is called the cart driver's seat (*Kutschersitz*): relaxed, bent slightly forward, the driver adapts to the movements of the horses while at the same time controlling them. This is different from the posture he takes when bringing the horses to a stop, tensing muscles and leaning back. Wikipedia notes,

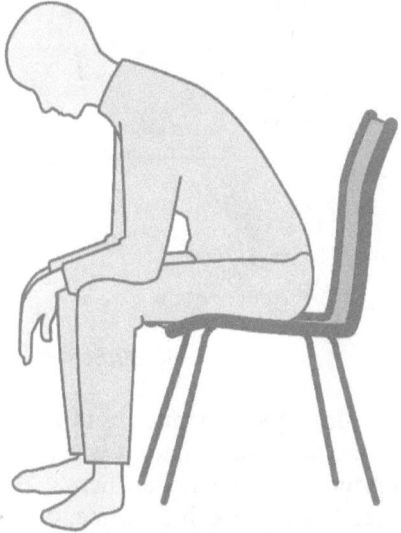

In nursing, physiotherapy, and medicine, the tripod position is a way of sitting that relieves or supports breathing. In the tripod position, the breathing area is increased by stretching the chest, which enables deep inhalation. The arms are supported on the legs and thus carry the weight of the shoulder girdle, from which the auxiliary respiratory muscles (including the pectoralis major) can expand the thorax and thus contribute to the breathing work otherwise essentially performed by the diaphragm.[6]

Fig. 38. The Tripod Position.

To undertake any form of breathing exercise, best adopt the tripod position and avoid the chest-out and belly-in posture. This is because the tripod position may appear soft and weak but—as it supports the organic structure of the organism while breathing—it is really quite strong. The breath is not only calmed, but also fundamentally strengthened and becomes a source of inner power and health.

On the other hand, if one yields to temptation and follows the Western ideal of uprightness, an essentially weak position is diluted by an apparent, external strength with the result that inner power cannot emerge. The trick is to move in the opposite way: straighten but without pulling the shoulder blades together; broaden the shoulders but without raising the breastbone. In other words, sit up in the tripod position and breathe freely.

---

[6] https://de.wikipedia.org/wiki/Kutschersitz (accessed 7/7/2022).

As Yang Chengfu puts it in his *Ten Basic Principles*: "Lifting the back means that the *qi* nestles against the back. If you hold your chest back, you naturally lift the back. If you lift the back, you shoot power out of your spine. Wherever you turn, there are no opponents" (2005).

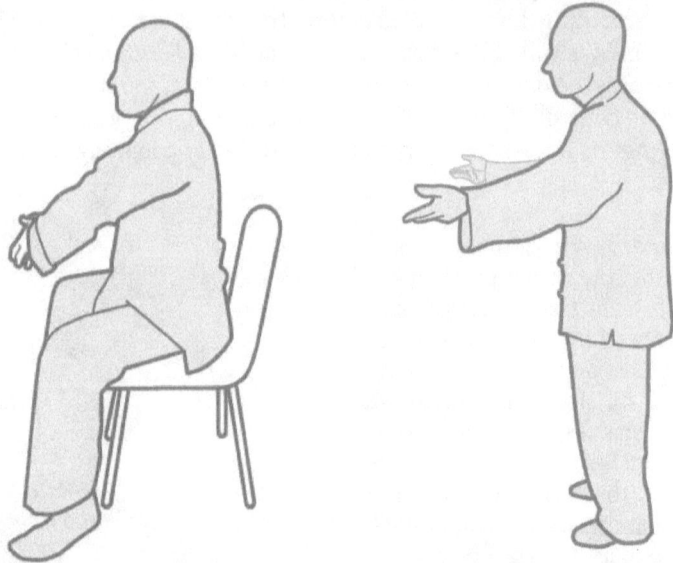

Fig. 39. Seated and Standing Qigong Practice.

In Qigong, as much as in Taiji, adepts transfer the slight forward bend of the torso, an apparent weakness that is key to the tripod position, into upright standing mode. Thereby they create the optimal conditions for the breath to flow freely and inner power to grow. Releasing the chest and opening the back, they enlarge the breathing area and stimulate the activity of the diaphragm.

Hao Yue-Rue (1877–1935), Wu/Hao-style Taiji master, states: "The chest must not be stretched, but should release downwards. The shoulders come together and move forward just a bit. This is called 'retaining the chest'" (Anders 2020). He continues to outline just how the subtle interplay of movement and breath works.

The Back

> Do not ask for a light burden, but ask for a strong back.
> —Franklin D. Roosevelt (1882-1945), US President

The *Süddeutsche Zeitung*, on November 22, 2016, reported: "Almost everyone has back issues. 70 percent of the German population suffer from back pain to a greater or lesser degree at least once a year. Many turn to their physician in hope for a cure. but when the back hurts, both patients and doctors often act incorrectly."[7]

Why do so many people have back problems? Partly because of wrong medical strategies. If there is pain in the lumbar spine, physicians strive to effect a cure right there. This may work for local injuries or inflammation, but more chronic and generic back pain has energetic causes. There is blocked *qi*-flow in the painful due to postural deficiencies. In Taiji terms, the connection between heaven and earth is cut.

Western medicine does not recognize this connection because it lacks the entire concept *qi*. As a result, physicians do not look at the whole person, instead searching localized causes and deviations from a norm in the smallest parts of the body. They trace any back pain to specific areas that are broken and work from there. Taiji adepts and Chinese doctors, on the other hand, hold a far-off view: as a microcosm of both body and universe, the back not only reflects conditions in the entire body but is also closely connected to the harmony of the cosmos.

It is thus not surprising the Western physicians usually find no direct cause when confronted with cases of chronically recurring back pain. As the *Süddeutsche Zeitung* points out, they as much as their patients tend to make the same four mistakes. First, about half the patients believe that they should see a physician if they have a back problem when in fact most issues are resolved by correcting the posture.

Second, patients insist on diagnosis and the use of equipment. 60 percent of those with insurance expect a detailed examination with complex imaging machinery; over two thirds even believe that the exact cause of their pain can be found with an X-ray, a CT scan, or an MRI. However, this is not true: physicians will not find anything with these tools.

Third, they rush to undergo diagnostic imaging before even trying physical therapy or other structural methods. This wastes insurance money and often leads to further unnecessary examinations and treatments.

Fourth and finally, physicians often give wrong advice, suggesting that patients stop moving. Scientifically, back rest is the best course of action when there is serious injury, such as a vertebral fracture or severe inflammation. Otherwise, the back should be moved to alleviate problems. However, many physicians recommend the opposite and thereby increase any pain and the subjective perception that the back is broken or worn out.

Chronic back pain is not an illness like any other, but the result of a slouched posture while walking. Human beings are designed to stand and walk upright, and "standing up straight" is not just a metaphor being determined and successful but also, in very concrete terms, indicates the lifelong

---

[7] www.sueddeutsche.de/gesundheit/rueckenkrankheit-aerzte-behandeln-ruecken schmerzen-oft-verkehrt-1.3260522 (accessed 7/7/22).

task to physically stand up. This does not happen by itself but has to be practiced. As long as people keep themselves upright, there will not be any back pain

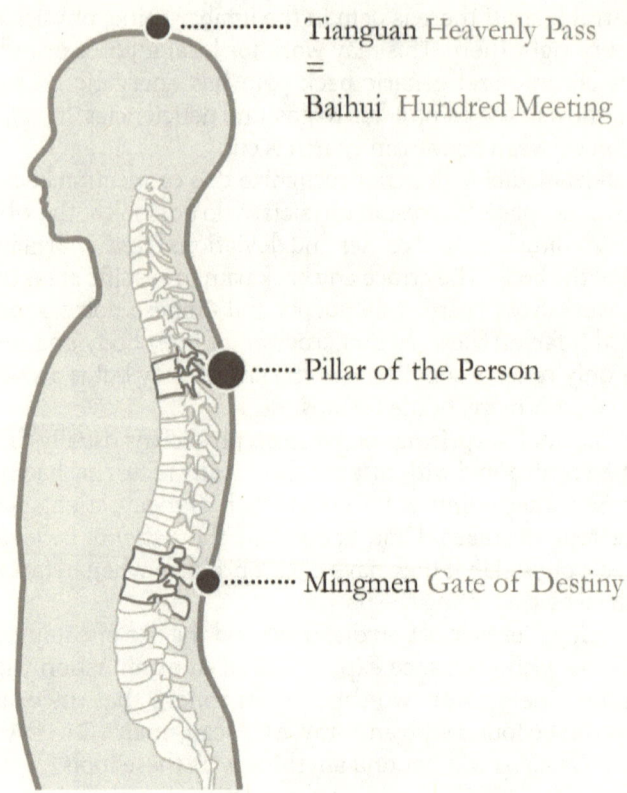

Fig. 40. Body Pillar and Gate of Life/Destiny.

Then again, naturally being upright does not mean pushing into a straight posture with artificial muscle tension. This only leads to stress and tightness, impacting especially the lumbar and cervical sections of the spine. Being upright and straight does not mean standing at attention, but positioning oneself calmly, with the head held high.

Taiji and Qigong teach us to function in this posture. Engaging with life courageously, adepts hold their head upright and never let it hang. They align the body on a straight axis between heaven and earth, allowing qi to flow freely, which makes the body feel good and elevates the mood. Sometimes back pain may be due to psychological issues, and even then, the practice helps by creating a better, uplifted attitude.[8]

---

[8] This has also been shown in a clinical study: http://taichiforhealthinstitute.org/the-first-tai-chi-for-back-pain-study/ (accessed 7/7/22).

The typical posture in Taiji and Qigong also works with an optimal adaptation to gravity. The spine is lifted, the center of gravity is low, both supported by the legs in such a way that the vertebrae are in the right place and can move freely. The slow movements of the form work through the entire body in a gentle manner, both challenging and protecting a damaged back. Consciously and mindfully guided by the attention, the movements carry the torso and limbs as if they were made of glass. All this is further enhanced by deep and conscious breathing, along the lines described in the Yang-family tradition.

Hands to Brain

> There is no animal more skilled with its fingers than man.
> —Yoshiya Hasegawa (b. 1966) Japanese physician

Wolfgang Höhn, my first Taiji teacher, translated an interesting book by the Japanese physician Yoshiya Hasegawa, entitled *Daumen-Yoga für das Gehirn* (Thumb Yoga for the Brain; 2019). A specialist for cognitive impairments, he shows how important the thumb is for the brain. Simple movement exercises for thumb and fingers improve blood flow to the brain and counteract Alzheimer's disease and dementia. If the fingers influence the brain, how important must the correct hand position be in Taiji?

When I started Taiji, I learned a relaxed form, a moving meditation that avoided physical exertion. Arms and hands, I was told, should be totally relaxed and move without muscle tension. As a result, my hands hung down like dead leaves on the limp branches of my arms. With no life of their own, they dangled from my wrists; quite loose and with no inherent tension, they

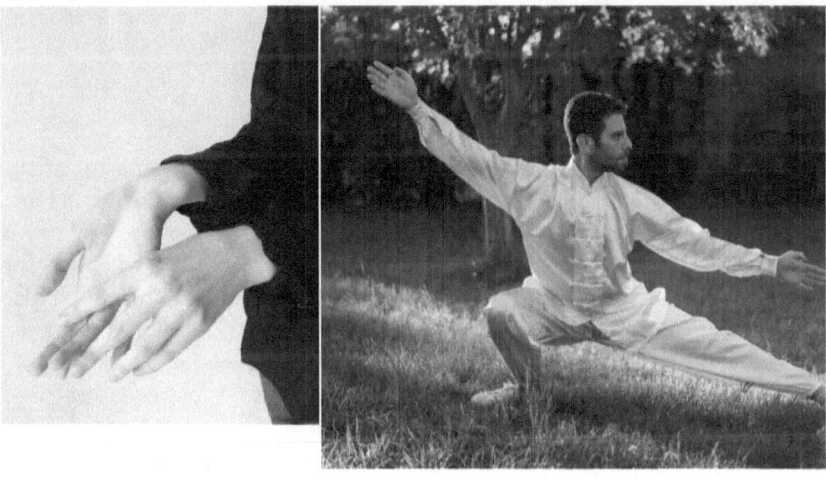

Fig. 41. Limp Hands and Tense Hands.

flowed wherever my arms moved. My Taiji looked like the movement of a dog on its hindlegs with its front paws hanging down.

This is still widespread in both Taiji and Qigong, an unfortunate feat because in this way brain and breathing are not stimulated. In the words of Master Chu, it is better to lie down on a couch to relax. Hands that just limp and formless are entirely unsuitable for Taiji.

On the far other extreme, there is also the opposite, that is, adepts stretch their fingers out straight and spread them apart to the point of almost being cramped. Such intense tension supposedly emphasizes the martial arts aspect of the practice. But this does not support for the breath, rather it blocks the flow of energy and tightens the mind.

Recent brain research shows that hand positions matter a great deal. Hasegawa in particular works with the homunculus diagram, developed by the Canadian neurosurgeon Wilder Penfield (1891-1976). This reveals just how much brain capacity individual sensory organs and body parts claim. The more brain capacity used for a body part, the larger it will be drawn.

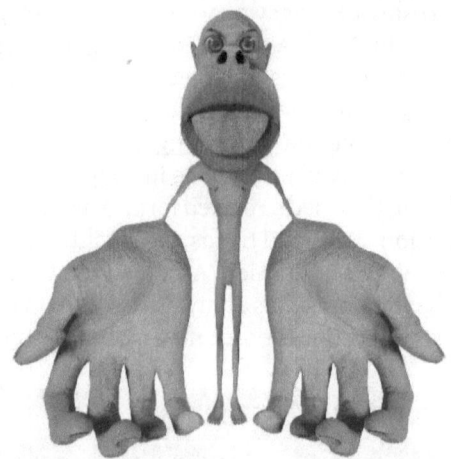

Fig. 42. The Humunculus Diagram.

It turns out that two thirds of the motor cortex and a quarter of the somatosensory cortex are responsible for the movement of the fingers and thumb alone. This means the hands work with two thirds of the brain area responsible for movement plus a quarter of its perceptual area. Thus, the homunculus has huge hands, much larger than the rest of the body. It also has thick lips, a fleshy tongue, and a good-size nose. These organs are responsible for the breath, the other key issue in Taiji and Qigong.

All this means that proper hand positions also affect breathing and thinking. The thumb is at the end of one of four so-called arm lines, defined by research on human connective tissue as linking muscles and fascia along the arms and back. One of these is the thumb line, which connects the thumb to the fourth rib. This means that the movements of the thumb directly influence the chest along this line. When I move my thumb, I affect my breathing.

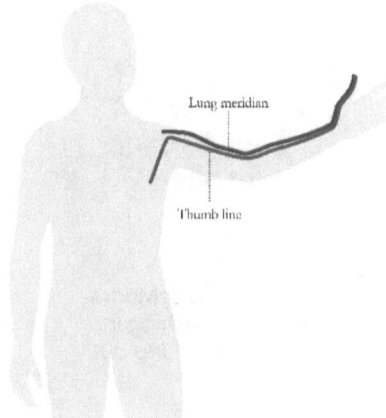

Fig. 45. Lung Meridian and Fascia Line.

This is also evident in Chinese medicine, which places the lung meridian roughly on the same line. Here, too, the thumb acts like a switch to activate the lungs.

I developed my Gate-of-Life Qigong, presented in *Das Qi verwurzeln* (2020), on the basis of these connections. In addition, my greater awareness of the hand-brain connection has also influenced the way I practice the Taiji form I have been committed to for over forty years. Many movements that were sort of fuzzy are now much clearer, giving expression to an amazing system with the thumb playing an essential role.

The hand in Taiji should be like an open tiger mouth: thumb and forefinger spread apart, as if you were to grab something with an open hand. The fingers remain relaxed, not rigidly stretched or spread out; they curve in slightly but rehre is some tension from the cupped hand that reaches for the void.

An almost equilateral triangle is formed between thumb, forefinger, and little finger; there is a straight fold of skin between thumb and forefinger, created by the loose tension between them.

If the hands join in tiger-mouth posture, they form a mudra that stimulates *qi* and regulates the breath, depending on type:

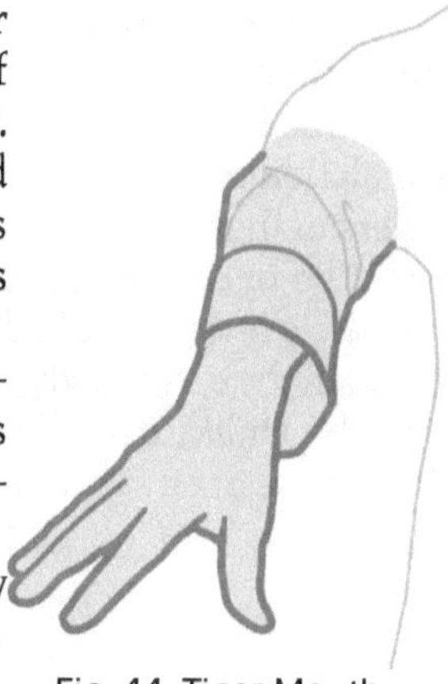

Fig. 44. Tiger Mouth.

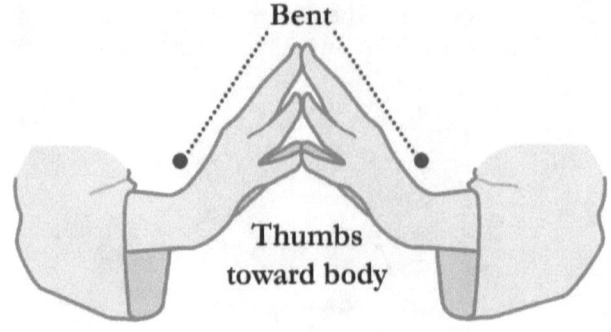

Fig. 45. Bent-wrist Mudra.
Inhalers – breathing in.
Exhalers – breathing out.

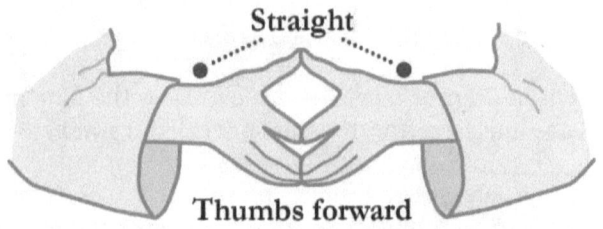

Fig. 46. Stretched-wrist Mudra.
Exhalers – breathing in.
Inhalers – breathing out.

Inhalers hold a mudra with bent wrists in their yin phase to support inhalation; exhalers assume the same position in their yang phase, that is, when they breathe out. Conversely, a stretched-wrist mudra supports the exhalation of the inhalers in their yang phase and the inhalation of the exhalers in their yin phase

The tiger mouth and mudra release the body tension that arises when the fascia lines in the body are stretched together. This kind of tension runs through the entire body; it has nothing to do with whether muscles are slack or tight. Unlike dead-leaf or pushed-out hands, which are part of external Taiji, these are a sign of inner power.

8
Breathing Types

Left-Handers and Inhalers

> I'll do that with my left hand!
> He has two left hands.
> —Figures of speech

Imagine you want to learn a new language, not to speak but also write. You sign up with a language school and take a course, but in the very first lesson they tell you that you must use a specific hand for writing: only the left! You are right-handed and always use your right hand to write; however, since you really want to learn this language and trust the teachers, you make an effort and practice writing with your left hand. You follow the rules and you do it, but it does not feel good at all.

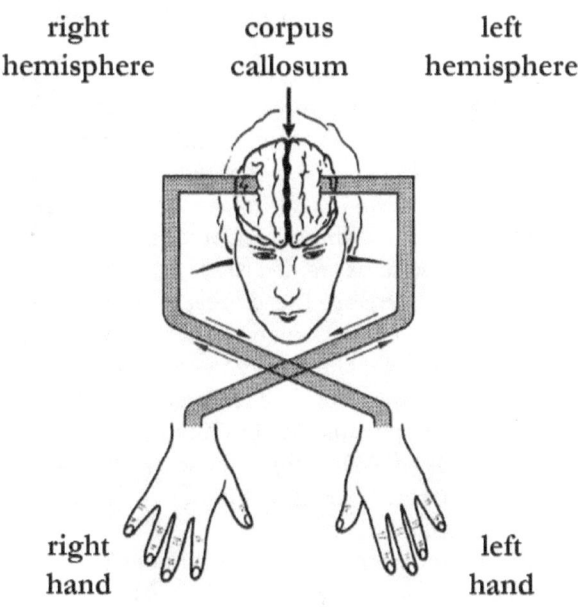

Fig. 47. Left and Right Hands in Relation to the Brain

This was the situation for left-handed children well into the 1970s. Since being right-handed was considered the norm, they underwent rigorous reeducation in early childhood, at the very latest by the time they started school. However, this retraining often caused problems: children had a hard time learning, their memory and speech were affected, and quite a few started to stutter, wet the bed, or became dyslexic. The psychological and cognitive damage was unknown at the time, and educators assumed they were doing them a favor since it was easier to live right-handed in a right-handed world. Today we know that handedness is an expression of the brain-hemisphere dominance and has nothing to do with being inept or of bad character. Nowadays both right- and left-handed people are equal, neither training to be like the other.

Still, there are other areas of life where different types are not recognized or treated as equal. A major area concerns breathing. For example, if you join a gym and start to work out, your trainer most likely will tell you to exhale upon exertion. However, the fact is that for some people it is easier and physiologically better to inhale upon exertion, which means they are taught a breathing technique that is entirely wrong for them. These inhalers are in the same situation as left-handers used to be, and it is high time that unique breathing types are recognized and accepted.

What, then, is a breathing type? The term does not refer to personal preference when breathing, that is, whether someone tends to breathe soft, shallow, or deep. It also has nothing to do with the activation the diaphragm or the chest.

What it means is that someone dominantly develops inner power when exhaling or inhaling. This is an inborn feature that cannot be changed. The entire body, not just the respiratory musculature, is shaped according to type. However, it is possible to overlay the natural type and develop habits that do not match it. Often well-meaning teachers, trainers, and therapists encourage people to adopt a wrong way of breathing, standing, or walking—just like left-handers used to be trained to act against their inborn nature.

It is not clear why there are these breathing types, just as we do not really know—although there are many theories—why some people are right-handed and others left. The fact remains that they exist and make a huge difference in the way people use their bodies. The technical term is "terlusollogy," coined by the musician Erich Wilk (1915-2000) and the pediatrician Charlotte Hagena (1909-2016). They work with one's date and time of birth: a more solar impact means one is an exhaler; a stronger lunar influence relates to being an inhaler.

One way to find out your type is to visit relevant websites.[1] Alternatively, you could see a trained terlusollogist or just observe yourself: make sure to breathe naturally and engage with what is most comfortable for you, avoiding any specific techniques and deliberate control of the breath that interfere with the natural flow. Your natural posture and movement patterns are revelatory. The bodies of exhalers tend to follow the downward

---

[1] Https://soluna.salix.in/allgemein/allgemein.html; https://atemformen.jimdo.com.

respiratory muscles and incline slightly forward when standing. Inhalers, on the other hand, are carried by the rising breath: they stand up straighter.

Once you know what your dominant type is, resist any form of retraining or moving in ways that are not comfortable. The culture tends to favor exhalers, which means that inhalers have a hard time catching their breath in the gym: inhalers who force themselves to exhale upon exertion against their natural breathing type gasp as a result. If they inhaled upon exertion, they would feel much better and have an easier time breathing.

Working against the breathing type over decades may well have similar consequences as the retraining of left-handers. Nobody has studied this systematically, but there is plenty of anecdotal evidence. Charlotte Hagena, who practiced this over forty years, reports many improvements when people started to go along with their breathing type (Hagena and Hagena 1997).[2] Speech therapists and voice coaches, too, report numerous successes as they work with the breathing types.

Self-Realization

> The aim of life is self-development. To realize one's nature perfectly—that is what each of us is here for.
> —Oscar Wilde (1854-1900), Irish writer

Teachers at my Taiji Academy have worked with the breathing types since 2006, making sure all positions and movements are adapted accordingly. While some people gain inner power upon exhalation, others draw strength from inhalation. Since this shapes the optimal posture of the body and the greatest ease in movement, adepts can feel their breathing type after some time. Standing and moving according to type feels right and is beneficial.

Still, it is not always easy to identify one's type since it can be overlaid by acquired habits: they are not natural but have been in place for so long that they feel normal. The improper use of body and breath over time causes the person to acquire the appearance and characteristics of the other type so that an inhaler who exhales upon exertion during work-outs after a while may well look like an exhaler.

Each type has prominent examples. Looking at celebrities—actors, musicians, athletes, politicians—it is usually easy to tell what breathing type they are, especially in people who work with their bodies. A typical inhaler was the dancer and choreographer Gene Kelly (1912-1996), best known for the film *Singin' in the Rain* (1952). Inhalers stand and move heel-to-toe because their pelvis and torso rest on the bones and joints of their legs for

---

[2] See also www.thieme-connect.de/products/ebooks/lookinside/10.1055/b-0039-172987 (accessed 7/8/22).

optimal inhalation. This results in an upright pelvic posture with stretched hip joints. The orientation is up, away from the earth.

A typical exhaler was the great dancer Fred Astaire (1899–1987), whose career in film, television, and theater spanned a total of seventy-six years. When walking, exhalers tend to supported themselves almost exclusively on the ball of the foot, cushioning the resulting forward fall with a spring, so that the body leans slightly forward. The slightly tilted pelvis hangs on the muscles and tendons of the legs while the hip joints are flexed. Jumping up, an exhaler looks quite different from an inhaler: to them it means getting back down to earth, not to defy gravity. Quite clearly, the energetic alignment toward the earth is reflected in Astaire's penchant for tap dancing.

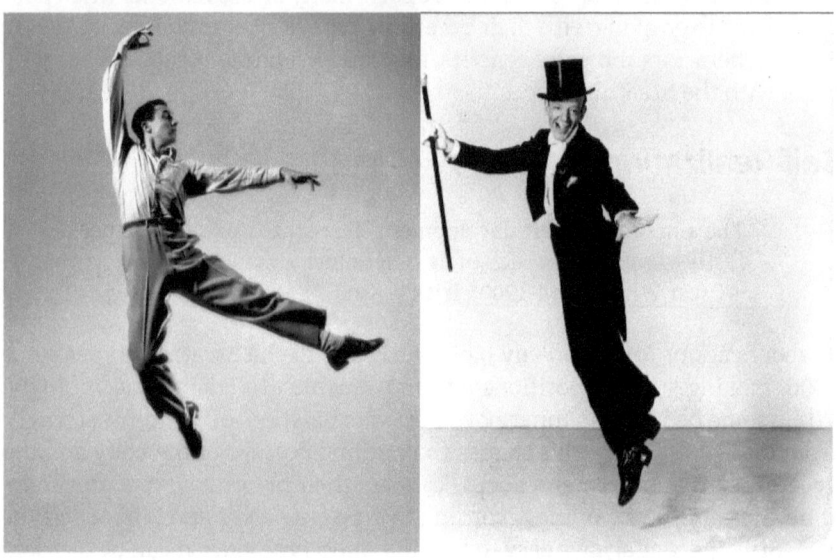

Fig. 48. Gene Kelly   and Fred Astaire

It is unlikely that Gene Kelly and Fred Astaire knew what breathing type they were, yet they intuitively mapped out their inherent faculties and used them to create their own coherent and distinctive artistic expression. The fascinating effect both have on the viewer—their inherent uniqueness—is rooted deeply in the realization of their own breathing preference and according adjustments. Both dancers realized their highest potential, developing themselves to the fullest.

The same applies in Taiji. Imitating the teacher's movements is likely to look silly or end up a parody, unless and until one makes them one's own and feels them from within. Ideally one finds a teacher of the same breathing type—which is what happened to me. Master Chu was of the same breathing type as myself, so that I was able to imitate him successfully. Had

I been an exhaler, most likely I would have given up, unable to realize my inner power, or moved on to find another master.

It takes a certain amount of courage as a teacher to allow the other breathing to express itself and nurture it properly. With Master Chu, everyone has to learn how to function as an inhaler—although he really should know better. His own teacher, Yang Shouzhong, was an exhaler and performed Taiji movements completely differently, as is obvious is the difference over the years.[3]

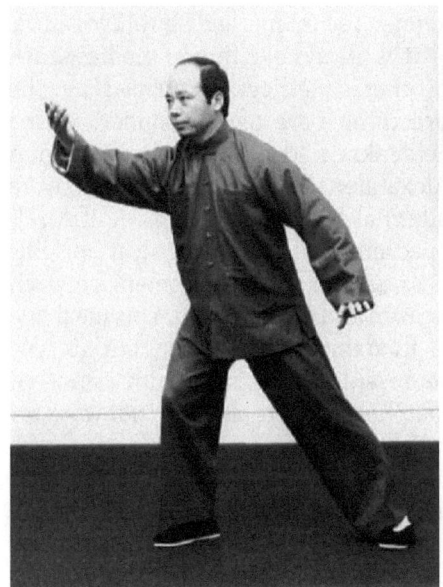
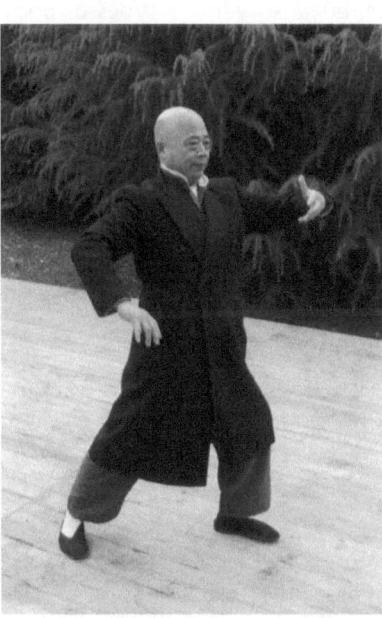

Fig. 49. Master Chu in 1984   and in 2022

Unfortunately, Master Chu misjudges both his own accomplishment— he developed an inhaler form of Taiji from an exhaler form— and that of his teacher when he claims that Yang Shouzhong intentionally disguised himself in the recordings. Yang's other students continue to preserve and teach his exhalation Taiji. As noted earlier, one particular development of this form in a lineage is now known as the Snake Style. Its representatives, like Master Chu, also claims to possess the only true Yang family form.

Claims to absolute truth are not helpful, here or elsewhere. Anyone who correctly recognizes his or her own disposition and works accordingly has most definitely not recognized that of all humankind. To appreciate that each and everyone has their own true disposition, different from those of others, is real wisdom and self-knowledge, coming much closer to the truth.

---

[3] See also www.youtube.com/watch?v=dj_Bt21Vdyo (accessed 8/3/22)

Half-Truths

> All truths are half-truths. To treat them as whole truths is to play the devil.
> —Alfred North Whitehead (1861-1947), British philosopher

Within its training program for teachers and course leaders, the Taiji Academy offers regular lectures that cover not only Taiji-related and Daoist topics, but also various types of bodywork, such as the Feldenkrais Method, Structural Integration (Rolfing), Alexander Technique, and Spiral Dynamics.

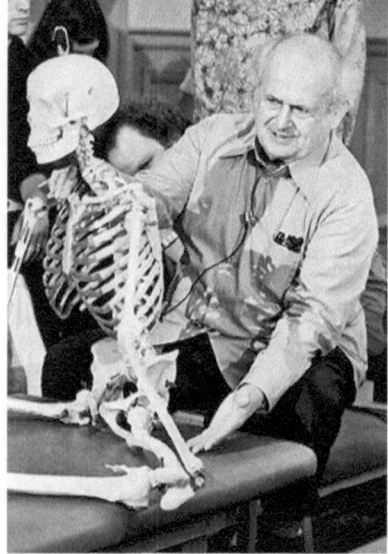

Fig. 50. Moshe Feldenkrais.

It is always exciting to see how each of these methods is shaped by the breathing type of its founder. Moshe Feldenkrais, Ida Rolf, Fredrick Matthias Alexander, and Christian Larsen were all exhalers. For example, Ida Rolf developed an ideal line of physical uprightness, similar to the alignment between heaven and earth in Taiji. This ideal line is fundamentally correct, but it only represents half the truth since it matches exhalers and does not work for inhalers.

Here is another example. Some time ago, I received a newsletter from the Center for Health, where Carina Rehberg reports on research by the naturopath Hans-Peter Greb on the correct way of walking. To him the only right way is by landing on the balls of the feet—anything different such as heel walking is of the devil.[4] Again this is a half-truth. Exhalers such as Dr. Greb walk on the ball of their feet, while inhalers step with their heel—an observation already true for infants taking their very first steps.

To me, this reveals a typical combination of great expertise and one-sided perspective. Dr. Greb (as much as other experts) considers only data that fit his preconceived notions, never even thinking about possible alternatives or opposites despite the fact that there are supporting data. Here is my open letter to him:

Dear Dr. Greb,

---

[4] www.zentrum-der-gesundheit.de/bibliothek/ratgeber/lebenshilfe/ballengang-ia (accessed 7/9/22)

The September 2015 newsletter of the Center for Health contains a detailed report on your view of the right way of walking, that is on the balls of the feet. It concludes in the same manner as it begins, with the statement, "The majority of the population walk on their heels and get sick from this. However, the original way of walking is on the balls of the feet."

To me, this is misleading and potentially harmful and I would like to correct it based on thirty-five years of Taiji experience and teaching. The fact is that only half of the people walk on the balls of their feet, while the other half walk on their heels. Which gait they prefer depends on their breathing type. Exhalers shift their weight to the front of the foot quickly after the heel hits the ground; inhalers emphasize heel contact and roll their feet.

Dear D. Greb, your own personal experience is most definitely true. But, in my opinion, you are incorrect when you generalize this personal experience and assume that it is the same for all people. Potential consequences are quite serious: if all people, independent of their breathing type, walk on the balls of their feet, most likely half of them will get sick.

I therefore ask you to look at the breathing type and invite you to include them as you do further research on the correct way of walking.

You will find that one group of people are indeed best suited to walking on the balls of their feet: these are the exhalers. However, even they do not just step with the forefoot but also make heel contact with the ground. I am deeply impressed by your high degree of body awareness. Based on your date and time of birth, you are completely solar, to a degree even where the sun made an extreme and unequivocal imprint on your life. This is quite and may explain why feel so strongly about ball walking and look at the types in such a one-sided way.

As helpful as your explanations may be for a better understanding of how exhalers function, you tend to take a subjective experience and make it into an objective truth. Based on my experience and convictions, gained especially over in the last ten years of Taiji work, I would like to make it very clear that there are always two truths about how a person aligns himself in the gravitational field, how he lies down, sits up, walks about, or operates in Taiji.

Dear Dr. Greb, please use my observations as food for thought and, if you please, join us at the Taiji Academy for an exchange. Breathing types can be an exciting and enriching approach for your project, opening your studies to the other half of humanity. Please do not hesitate to contact me.

Best regards,

Frieder Anders

The Alphorn Player

> Music is the most beautiful of all sounds.
> —Théophile Gautier (1811-1872), French writer

During a recent training in the Alsace, everything went wonderfully well: the weather, the hotel, the food, and the course *qi* were excellent. One of the participants was Fritz Frautschi, an alphorn player and terlusollogy specialist from Switzerland.[5] He agreed to give us a demonstration, and we all, including myself, were deeply struck by the power of the instrument: it made a beautiful sound, rich, yet light and very soothing.

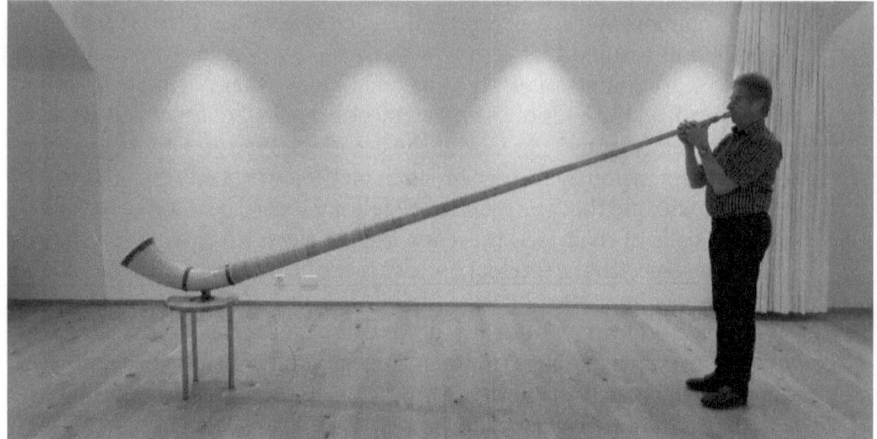

Fig. 51. Fritz Frautschi.

Here, too, the breathing type comes into play. Fritz is an inhaler who has to stand with a lift in the pelvic area, a rather difficult feat when playing the alphorn. The horn can be up to twelve feet long and is placed on the ground, which creates a gradient that causes the player, almost automatically, to assume a slightly inclined, oblique posture.

This posture is the hallmark of the exhaler. The muscles responsible for exhaling lift the tailbone and bring the pelvis into that slightly forward tilt that solidifies in the physique. Inhalers, on the other hand, show a more pronounced musculature involved in inhalation and they tend to straighten the pelvis and stretches the hip joints.

Fritz had practiced the alphorn for years with a posture that contradicted his breathing type. He stood like an exhaler even though he is an in-

---

[5] www.alphornatelier.ch (accessed 7/9/22).

haler. As a result, he developed abdominal pain, since the abdominal muscles while blowing the alphorn work very hard but he was not using them correctly. His body showed him his erroneous ways by manifesting pain. Knowing about the breathing types, he went to the Mannheim physician Christian Hagena, the husband of Charlotte, for help who in turn referred him to a knowledgeable wind-instrument teacher. He duly taught him how to adopt the correct playing position for his breathing type.

To adjust to his breathing type, Fritz Frautschi came up with a simple but effective trick: he constructed a stool to rest his alphorn. This raise in position decreased the angle of inclination, allowing the player to change his posture. Fritz was able to stand upright as an inhaler and blow his horn more smoothly: his physical ailments disappeared.

Breathing Naturally

> Always keep your arms and legs rounded,
> then you will never exhaust yourself.
> —Taiji Classic

From time to time, articles appear on the internet that teach people how to improve their breathing, but they tend to spread the same clichés. An example is the article, "How to Get More Air While Breathing," by Beate Splett and Annett Böhm in the blog of the Mitteldeutscher Rundfunk radio station, dated June 10, 2021.[6]

It presents the breathing process as a mere physical mechanism that can be controlled by the will. Again, this is only a half truth: breathing is an autonomous function of the human body and happens automatically. The respiratory center is in the brainstem, from where muscles, organs, and cells are supplied with oxygen with every breath—quite without consciously control. Due to this automation, we can continue to breathe (and live) when not fully conscious, during sleep or when unaware in everyday life.

On the other hand, breathing is the only autonomous bodily function we can influence intentionally, at least for a time. This makes the use of breathing techniques possible. However, caution is advised, for it is all too tempting to overestimate the power of the will. Breathing is not a mechanical part of a body machine that we can control completely. It contains a significant measure of self-regulation. This means that the Rundfunk presentation is full of clichés, pretending that breathing is nothing more than a mechanical inflation of the pulmonary sacs through regular movements.

---

[6] www.mdr.de/ratgeber/gesundheit/atmung-luftnot-atemtechniken-100~amp.html?utm_medium=referral&utm_source=upday (accessed 7/9/22)

The blog gives a series of tips that are a sheer nightmare for any Taiji practitioner, beginning with its insistence on the best posture as being with chest out, shoulders back, and arms up or back. Such a stiff and rigid posture with contracted shoulder blades, in fact, narrows the breathing space and does not help at all. Another piece of advice is that one should always breathe deeply into the belly and breathe everything out just as consciously. This again is not true and the fact is that the body—depending on the breathing type—releases air (inhaler) or sucks it in (exhaler) of its own accord. Plus, it is quite impossible to breathe deeply into the abdomen with the chest pushed out and the shoulders pulled back. Nor is this healthy for every breathing type.

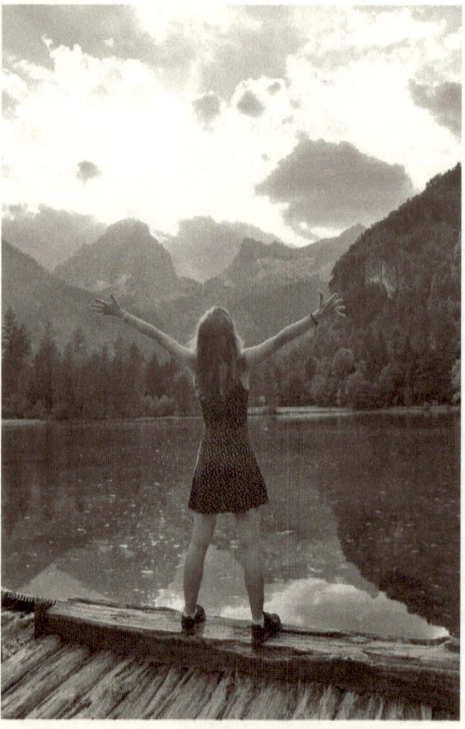

Fig. 52. The Common but Wrong Posture for Deep Breathing.

Then again, the authors emphasize breathing into the side body, which is not bad, but they make no mention of diaphragmatic breathing despite the fact that the diaphragm actually does the main work in the breathing process. Eventually, the article culminates in the suggestion to undertake an exhalation exercise on a regular basis that looks somewhat like the illustration above (Fig. 52). It says, "To enhance the exercise, stretch out both arms and reach toward the ceiling: this is a wonderful stretch for long periods in the office!" It may well have benefits, but is certainly not relaxing.

If you keep your arms stretched up, you will quickly run out of breath. The ancient Romans already knew that: they crucified people with their arms raised. They could then no longer breathe out and suffocated painfully.

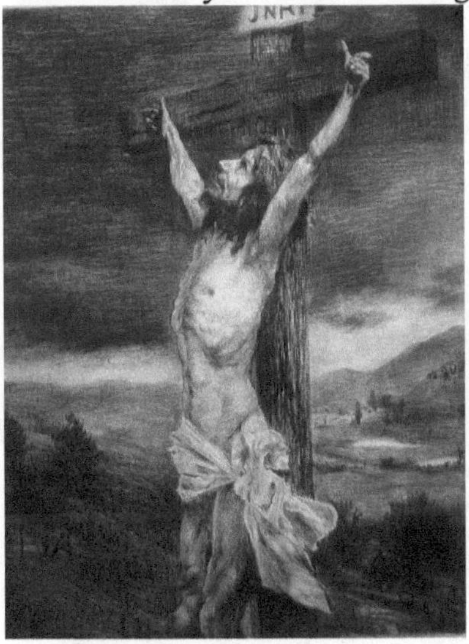

Anatomically, the process of crucifixion is not hard to explain. The large pectoral muscle is attached to the ribs and has an insertion in the upper arm. Moving the arm inward from here expands the lungs and aids inhalation. During crucifixion, the lungs no longer have the opportunity to return from this activating position to a relaxing exhalation. Body weight and arms stretched sideways and up prevent movement of the pectoral muscle. The condemned can no longer breathe. So, beware of any non-moving breathing exercises—they may have unwanted side effects.

Fig. 53. The Crucifixion of Christ.

Pelvic Breathing

In Taiji we breathe less with the chest muscles than from the pelvis. More precisely, we activate the diaphragm indirectly through movements that emanate from the pelvis. Of course, we cannot directly sense the diaphragm, since it has no neural connections. This means we have no direct access to it and no awareness of its activity.

So what can we do for the diaphragm? First of all, we need to adopt the right posture. We must round our backs and under no circumstances pull our shoulders back as during crucifixion. This opens the lungs and allows room for the breath to flow freely. When seated, it happens best in the tripod position. Next, the most effective movement to activate the diaphragm comes from in the pelvis or, more precisely, the lumbar spine. Here originates the deepest breath, the "true breath" in Taiji—in an energy center the Chinese call Gate of Life or Destiny (*mingmen*).

The word *ming* means "command" or "order." By extension it indicates the will of heaven, an imperial decree, and personal destiny, including a preordained life expectancy. The character *men* literally means "gate," "door," or "opening." It appears in many Chinese terms and always denotes an unimpeded entrance or exit.

According to traditional Chinese body cosmology, the original vitality of the human being is anchored in the Gate of Life. Confucians describe it as the Taiji or Great Ultimate of the body as a microcosm of the universe, while Daoists call it "the gorge of mysterious origins." It is located in the lower back area, near the kidneys, that is where the diaphragm attaches to the spine. In gastronomy (related to beef or veal), these pillars are known as "kidney cones."

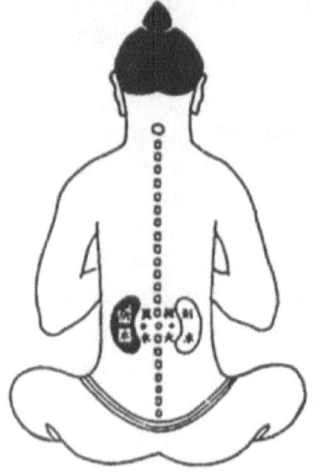

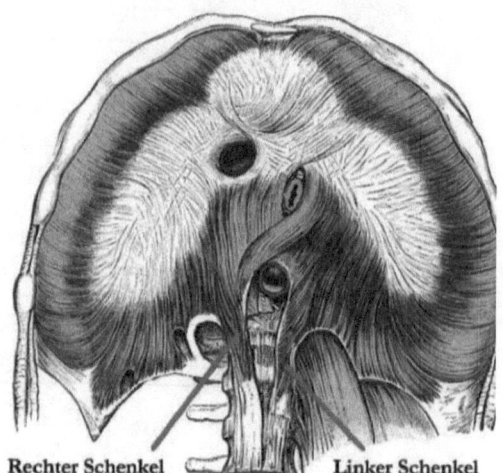

Fig. 54. The Gate of Life.   Fig. 55. The Pillars of the Diaphragm.

Movements of the lumbar spine or pelvis pull on these pillars or cones and tighten or loosen the diaphragm. Which means that as by moving the Gate of Life, Taiji trains the respiratory strength of the diaphragm and does not use the auxiliary muscles of the abdomen as taught in other breathing techniques. This indirect method allows people to be breathed by the body and thus opens access to the direct respiratory muscles.

Breathing like this is new for the body and takes practice to learn. However, the reward is well worth the effort. Breathing with the Gate of Life opens practitioners to working with "true breath." It is both stimulating and relaxing at the same time, meditative and active in equal measure. My own Qigong form called Gate-of-Life Qigong offers an introduction to this in theory and practice (see Anders 2020). Take a deep breath and do not crucify your diaphragm.

9

True Inner Power

The Coffee Maker

Around 1981, my long-term teacher, Master Chu, first visited my school in Frankfurt. At the time, my students and I had been studying Taiji for five years: we were still highly idealistic, often worked in dungarees, and had long hair hanging in our faces.

Master Chu amazed us with some unexpected statements. For example, he compared people doing Taiji to a car: the arms and legs are the wheels, the center is the engine, the *qi* is the fuel, and the spirit is like the spark that gets everything going, the electricity from the battery. Some were downright shocked by this analogy. They had started Taiji to get to know their body as a holistic organism, not as a well-oiled machine as it is presented in Western medicine. But if you consider that everything a person envisions is a reflection of his or her inner world of experience and position in the world, then Master Chu's analogy maybe was not so bad.

With that in mind, I would now like to take a closer look at the motor of the Taiji movement machine. Instead of a car, I prefer the coffee maker as an analogy, that is, a fully automated espresso maker complete with grinder. First, it grinds the beans into a powder, then it mixes this with pressurized hot steam. Through this process, the raw materials water and ground beans are transformed into a nobler liquid. The result is a delicious espresso, a true elixir of life that makes you happy.

Something similar happens in Taiji. It starts with natural *qi*, the life energy that everyone has in varying amounts over the course of life. Under pressure of the diaphragm, this energy is mixed with the *qi* inhaled as breath and is refined. The result is a new level of delicious *qi*, like espresso a true elixir of life that makes you happy.

According to Chinese medicine and Daoism, the center where the *qi* collects is the lower elixir field (*dantian*), an energy vortex located two to three finger breadths beneath the navel. It connects to an acupuncture point on the surface of the belly, but the center is deep inside. In the Indian system, it matches the chakra known as *manipura*, "Shining Jewel," associated with volition, power, personality, and wisdom. At the same level on the back, the lower elixir field opens near the kidneys at the point where the pillars of the diaphragm attach to the lumbar spine. This is an area well known for herniated disks: the Chinese think of it as the Gate of Life.

86 / Chapter 9

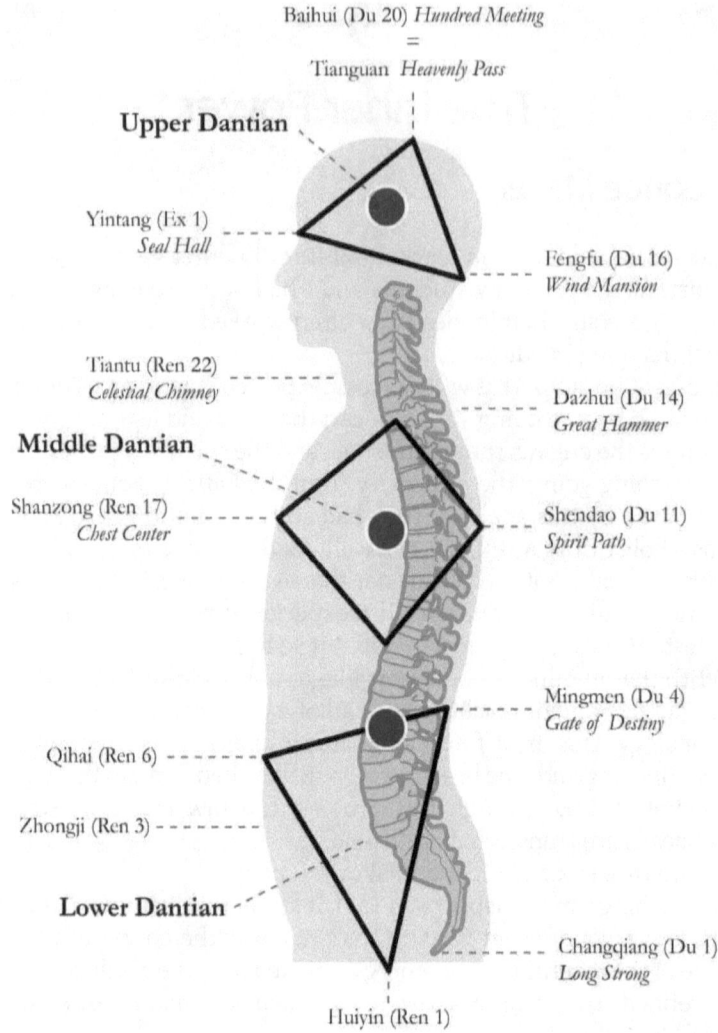

Fig. 56. Three Elixir Fields with Gate of Life/ Destiny.

At the Taiji Academy, we have studied the Gate of Life and its connection to the diaphragm for many years. Working with breathing types, we found that moving lower spine allows the are below the Gate of Life to open and close, thereby setting the true breath in motion like a pump. This does not come about through voluntary activation of the respiratory muscles, but happens involuntarily. The movement of the back moves the pillars of the diaphragm so that breathing happens in the same way as during sleep: it breathes us. The research resulted in the development of Gate-of-Life Qigong (Anders 2020), a good way to activate the true breath.

To return once more to the analogy, *qi* as biological raw material assembles in the lower elixir field like ground coffee beans come to rest in the coffee maker. Just like the grounds are then mixed with steam, so *qi* is activated by the breath, pressurized and moved through the body like a pure elixir of life. The motions of the steam in the coffee maker match the spinal movements in the Gate of Life area. This is a truly alchemical process: ti refines the body into vital, cosmic breath.

It is cosmic because it does not come from us but originates in a higher, more universal sphere. Spirit is the agent who guides the grinding and steaming process: it creates inner power as well as inspiration. And how, let me ask, could people ever have invented a fully automated coffee maker without knowing this process from their own body?

Expansion of Consciousness

> Paradise is barred and the cherub behind us.
> We have to make the trip around the world and see
> If it is open again perhaps somewhere in back.
> —Heinrich von Kleist (1777-1811), German poet and playwright

A few years ago, the German news magizine *Der Spiegel* (2017/26) published an article entitled "The Third Eye." It was about a failed attempt at expanding consciousness with the help of a new synthetic drug. As it turned out, the substance contained one or more unknown ingredients that caused horrific experiences in the participants. They called the local fire brigade who were amazed, thinking, "What kind of idiots are these guys?" The group included physicians, naturopathic doctors, homeopathic healers, and yoga teachers, that is, practitioners of various backgrounds dedicated to using gentle healing methods without the supposedly toxic drugs produced by the pharmaceutical industry.

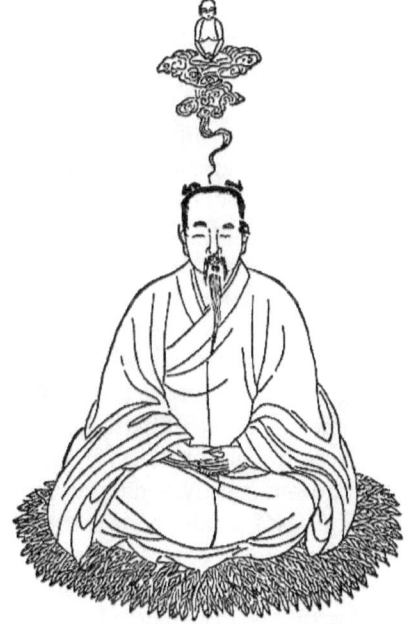

Fig. 57. The Immortal Embryo Emerges

And here they all were, embroiled in a horrific altered state induced by synthetic drugs!

Such scenarios are not uncommon. The European cultural TV channel Arte once ran a report about the charismatic and enterprising Indian guru Osho, better known as Rajneesh. Prominent in the 1970s, he assembled large numbers of followers both in India and the US. He promised self-knowledge and expansion of consciousness, then skillfully manipulated them, utilizing their hope to attain enlightenment.

Being of the same generation myself, I was never tempted to join a cult. On the other hand, I had my own awakening experience in 1970, when I was part of a New York theater group. I, too, felt the draw of the consciousness-expansion movement. Great was the regressive longing to be able to dive back into the paradise conditions of a childlike, harmonious relationship with the entire world. The longing for such love is still around today. It leads to drug and alcohol abuse or even to those supposedly consciousness-expanding experiments described in the magazine.

People engaging in these activities are motivated by a strong desire to return to the origin. They believe they can find it in a different place, a paradise where the ego no longer exercises control. However, they can never succeed because they fail to recognize the basic conditions of human existence. In fact, their regressive fantasies are based on a thorough misunderstanding of human nature: they cannot accept that we are beings determined by both having a body and being a body.

Their idealized vision of the expansion of consciousness goes back to a critique of the dominant Western understanding that we have a body, understood to be at the root of all manner of bodily exploitation, the way of using it like a tool that is geared to perform in a certain way. Instead of this performance body, they are looking for a completely different physical experience, a flow in which consciousness dissolves. In pure sensuality, they hope to be all body. But in fact, this self-dissolution is one-sided and limited. Only the interlocking of both, having a body and being a body, is holistic.

Taiji provides is a way to unite and integrate both. Here the mind is awake, not foggy or ecstatic, and with its help we learn and perform the movements. Awake mindfulness is the way of expanding consciousness engendered in Taiji practice: it does not subject the body to sheer will power but guides it, gently and wisely, to movements that arise as if of their own. Mindfulness includes feeling the body in the practice, listening to it and respecting its impulses. This creates a conscious flow that opens the person to a completely different kind of spontaneous freedom: the experience of practiced activities taking on a life of their own. Here is where we find the unity of being and having.

The Taiji path is much more difficult than taking a pill, sinking into intoxication, and regressing to a preconscious state. But it is a true path to selfhood and offers a powerful expansion of consciousness.

The Diamond

> Runes are old Germanic writing symbols. The collective term includes characters from different alphabets in different temporal and regional uses.[1]

Late fall, when the days get shorter and darkness comes earlier, is also the time when Germans remember their dead, notably on the Day of the Dead and Memorial Day in early November. These festivals go back to ancient Celtic and Germanic practices.

Another important feature of Nordic culture is the writing system of runes, used in Iceland until the late Middle Ages. The name "rune" derives from the root *rún* (Gothic *rūna*), which literally means "mystery." In modern German, it is retained in words like *raunen* and *Geraune* (murmur). Each rune symbolizes a letter but also contains a metaphorical and spiritual meaning, hiding a secret of its own.

The one most relevant rune in this context is called *Ing*. Adopting the name of the main fertility god, it denotes a nasal "n," the sound found in the suffix *-ing* or or *-ung*. It takes the form of a diamond, whose spiritual meaning is inner fire: "Ing symbolizes the spark of creation, the power to give life and make the land fertile. The inner fire drives every human being toward spiritual fulfillment. It gives us strength even in difficult times. This fire can lie dormant for many years; but once we discover it, it is almost impossible to erase. Ing teaches that the past cannot be changed: we can only affect the present."[2]

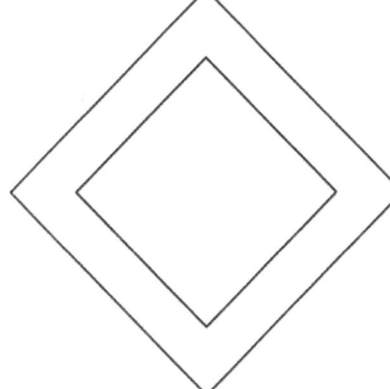

Fig. 58. The Rune *Ing*.

The diamond shape has a notoriety of its own: the German chancellor Angega Merkel tended to hold her hands in that position—maybe aware of its deeper symbolism, maybe not. In addition, in a slightly modified form, with lines intersecting, it has become a major sign in the digital world, here known as hashtag (#).

---

[1] https://de.wikipedia.org/wiki/Runen (accessed 7/10/22).
[2] www.runenkunde.de (accessed 7/10/22).

The real secret of the diamond is that it is an important form element in the human body. The inner fire symbolized by *Ing* in the Germanic runes corresponds to the life energy *qi*. If we use our arms and legs—not just the hands—to form a diamond when standing of moving, the inner fire of *qi* flows freely and burns brightly. The diamond, that is, has a magical quality, just like the runes.

How do we get to this magic diamond in Taiji? The basis is initially formed by two triangles as shown in Fig. 59. At the very center is the acupuncture point Du 12 on the Go. Called "body pillar" or "pillar of the person" (*shenzhu*), it is located on the back between the third and fourth thoracic vertebrae, opposite the solar plexus. If we hold both arms out so that the elbows are at this level, the line from elbow to elbow goes right through the body pillar and forms the base of the upper triangle.

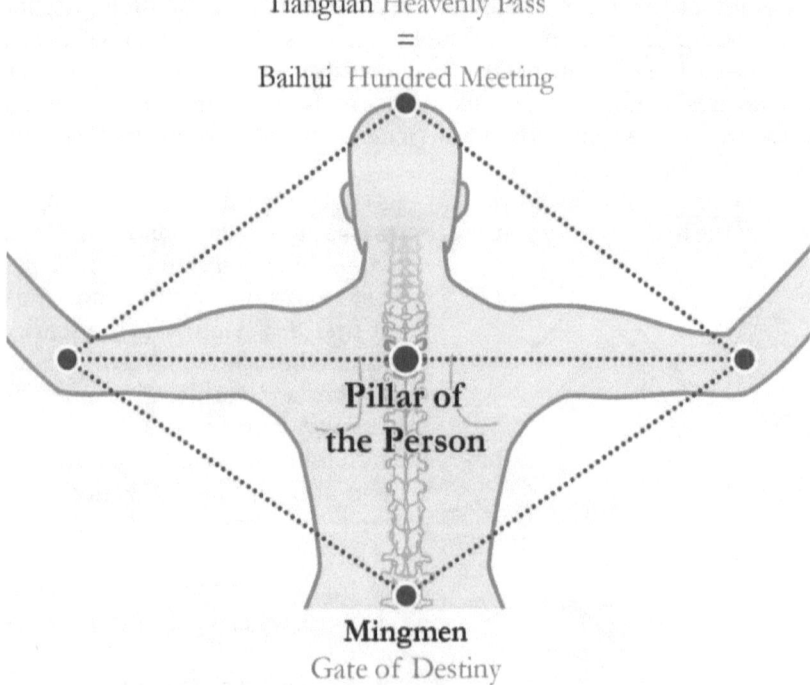

Fig. 59. Two Triangles Make up the Diamond.

Its tip is at the top of the head (Du 20), known as Baihui (Hundred Meeting) or Tianguan (Heavenly Gate). It is in a straight vertical line above the body pillar. The tip of the lower triangle is the Gate of Life, right below it. Together they form the magic diamond of Taiji movements.

In order to activate the flow of *qi* with the diamond, it is necessary to adopt the basic Taiji posture. The upper arms float at chest level, that is, in line with the central elixir field, and form a solid unit with the shoulder girdle. This keeps the outer edges of the triangle stable. At the same time, the shoulder blades should be flat on the back so they do not stick out. This causes the thoracic spine to rise and the back to round. In this manner the body pillar pushes outward as a noticeable knob and is activated while breath rushes down the back.

In order to activate the tip of the upper triangle, it is imperative that the head remains erect. In exhalers, it tips slightly forward and feels as if its top is lifted by a cord tied to the crown of the head. In inhalers, the chin is raised a bit, striving more actively toward the sky yet without straining the neck. These features were well known to the old masters. The second of Master Yang Chengfu's *Ten Basic Principles* is: "Hollow the chest and straighten the back" (*hanxiong babei*).[3]

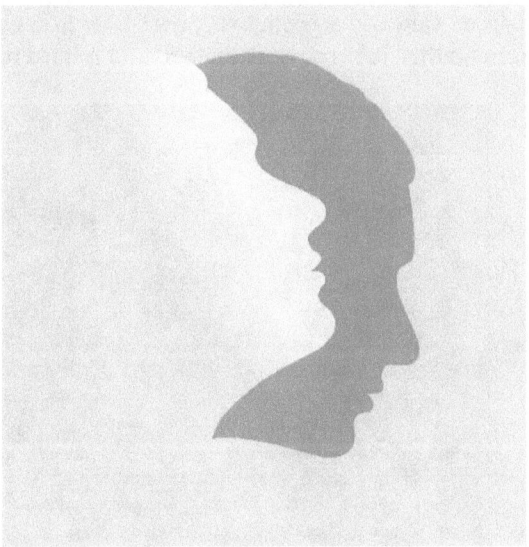

Fig. 60. Head Positions of Inhalers, Exhalers

It may sound bit cryptic or weird, but in fact refers to lifting the body pillar without letting the chest area sinking in. Rather, the elbows extend outward, bringing the shoulder blades into a flat position. The back should be slightly rounded and the body pillar activated at all times. If this is maintained throughout Taiji and Qigong practice, the "power comes from the

---

[3] www.daniel-roga.de/taijiquan-tai-chi-chuan-theorie-prinzipien/10-prinzipien-von-yang-cheng-fu.html (accessed 7/10/22).

spine," as the classics have it. Such is the deeper meaning and practical application of key symbols such as the diamond.

Mars and Venus

> How sweetly she climbs over dung
> And I've never even kissed her!
> —Martin Luserke (1880-1968), German educator and writer

This line is from a rather grotesque knightly play by Martin Luserke, called *Blood and Love*. Full of chivalry and love magic, it is still popular with German amateur theater groups. I know it well because I acted in a teenage production in 1960.

The performance had its very own charm: all roles were male; the stage design was hand-crafted and hand-painted. I played the gruff knight Wolf von Wolfseck with a beard made from my own hair: I had picked up cut tresses at the barber's and stuck them to my then beardless cheeks with glue. I do not recommend this: it burns horribly hell and is hard to remove.

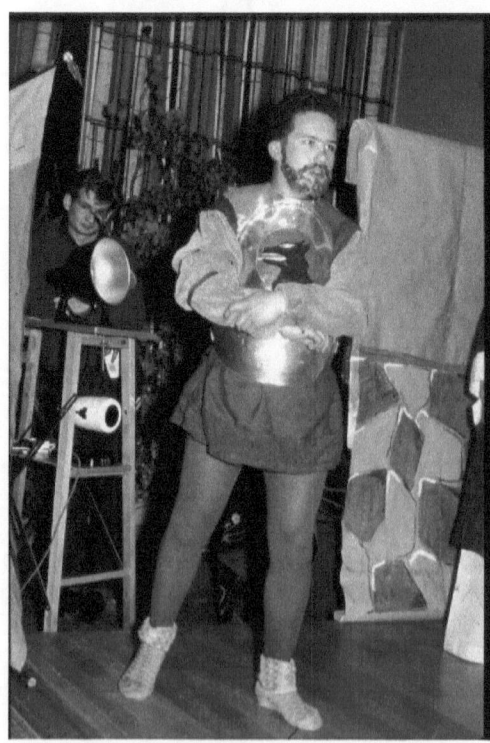

Fig. 61. Frieder Anders, 1960.

The play ends with almost everyone dead because they mistake a deadly poison for a love potion. Its central theme of love and war reflects the primal principles of Mars and Venus, core issues of life everywhere, expressed in key questions such as: How do I assert myself? How do I differentiate myself? How can I give and receive love without losing myself in the other or having to force myself to assert myself? We have to reconcile the energies of these two primal principles of Mars and Venus if we want to lead a fulfilling life.

What, then, might this reconciliation look like? In the afterword to the German translation of the book *King, Warrior, Magician, Lover* (1990), Rüdiger Dahlke writes:

> Almost all educators and even some founders of religions recommend, preach, and demand not of reconciliation with the original principle of Mars but with its opposite pole, Venus....
>
> It is always easiest to simply demand the opposite, but as we see everywhere, it just does not work. Taking action against violence with love has little chance of success in the long run. (2014, 245)

Dahlke puts it in a nutshell: one must not suppress the warrior within. All too often the apparent peacefulness of do-gooders is not real love, but a way to repress and deny the Mars principle. It presents a morality that prevents autonomy, the state that develops "from the possibilities of the unhindered experience of one's own perceptions, feelings, and needs," as the psychoanalyst Arno Gruen puts it (1990, 11). By doing so, one does not prevent the evil that such people want to prevent, but becomes a source of evil oneself.

In Taiji, we have the chance to reconcile Mars and Venus, more so than in the religions of compassion and slave morality. In a way, the two are like yin and yang: one principle wants to fight, the other does not—and in a certain sense, Taiji does both. It does not suppress aggression, but transforms it into an inner power that is victorious but will not hurt the opponent. Inner power both fights the opponent and does not fight at the same time. The way of the warrior consists of learning skills that could destroy another, but at the same time the ideal is never to have to use those skills. It works with a dangerous love or lovable dangerousness in dealing with the opponent.

Properly understood, Taiji is not a gentle martial art that only caresses the opponent with its movements—too much Venus and not enough Mars. Nor is it an aggressive martial art that only strikes with brute force—too much Mars and not enough Venus. Rather it joins, unites, and integrates the two principles in the growth of inner power, which requires the careful nourishing of *qi* as well as physical and mental self-cultivation.

You learn to fight just to be able to defend yourself. But this does not stop with the acquisition of merely external techniques and skills. The true method of Taiji lies in the cultivation of the whole human being. Through years of practice, the body becomes strong and elastic, like a ball that cannot be defeated with brute force. The arms become, as Yang Chengfu puts it in the sixth of his *Ten Basic Principles*, like "iron wrapped in cotton,"[4] although during practice they are only moved lightly and in a relaxed way.

The movements intertwine in sometimes barely visible spiral movements, allowing head, legs, core, and spine to become rotating segments of a round body that simultaneously attracts and repels an attack, like a tornado. And because the body is governed by the mind, the body becomes "spiritual," which makes Taiji a spiritual practice. As Wu Yuxiang says in the Taiji classics, "If you direct all movements through the mind, your ordinary physical strength is transformed into spiritual energy. Then your movements will no longer be clumsy and sluggish" (Anders 2003, 142).

Thus, the highest power of defense develops and both principles, fighting and non-fighting, are reconciled.

The Flood-like Qi

> Sleep for eight hours each night to be well rested and fit for the day. During sleep, the body releases many substances that strengthen the immune system. In addition to healthy sleep, it is also important to avoid stress. The body's internal stress hormones, such as adrenaline, temporarily overload the organism and the number of immune cells decreases. Build enough relaxation into your everyday life, so the body has more energy left for the immune system.
> —TK Home Solutions website[5]

"Flood-like *qi*" is an expression of the Chinese philosopher Mencius (Mengzi), who lived around 370-290 BCE. Human beings in his view are both selfish and altruistic. They have an inborn nature that is essentially good but is lost or overlaid through external influences and circumstances. Sleep regenerates it to a certain extent but not completely. Beyond that, it has to be cultivated and relearned through regular practice. The book *Mengzi* records the following dialogue:

---

[4] https://taiji-forum.de/taichi-taiji/taiji-klassiker/zehn-wesentlichen-gebote (accessed 7/10/22).
[5] https://homesolutions.tkelevator.com/de-de/ratgeber/magazin/fit-und-gesund/staerken-sie-ihr-immunsystem/ (accessed 7/10/22).

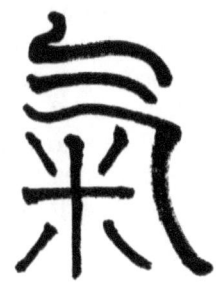

Fig. 62. Qi.

A disciple asked, "May I ask what you mean by 'flood-like qi'?"

Mencius said, "It is hard to explain. It is a form of *qi* as vast and firm as it can be. If you nurture it by straightforward action and never impair it, then it fills all between heaven and earth. Doing so, *qi* is a companion to righteousness and Dao; without this, it will starve. It is generated through the long accumu-lation of righteous acts and not something that can be seized through a single good deed. If, in your actions, there is any sense of inadequacy in your heart, it will starve. . . .

The task of nurturing this *qi* must never be forgotten by the heart, but you must not meddle and try to help it grow. Do not be like the simpleton from Song. He was so concerned that the sprouts in his field were not growing well that he went and tugged at each one. He went home utterly exhausted and said, "Oh, I've made myself ill today! I've been out helping the sprouts to grow." His sons rushed out to look and found the stalks all shriveled up. (2A2; Eno 2016, 40)

This story appears variously in ancient literature and most likely was part of the general wisdom of the people. It is still highly relevant today and even appears in a contemporary proverb: "Pulling on sprouts to help them grow" (*bamiao zhuchang*). In essence, it expresses the principle of nonaction: if you do too much, you ruin everything.

The Chinese term for nonaction is *wuwei*, two characters that can be read as an imperative: "Do not intervene!" A central principle in Daoism, it states that one must never interfere with the autonomous processes of natural becoming, since any active intervention will have a destructive effect. The restraint and gentle handling of both animate and inanimate nature (as well as of oneself), however, is in itself quite active, encompassing an attitude of cultivation and patience, waiting until things develop by themselves. The *Daodejing* says: "Do not intervene and there is nothing that is not done" (ch. 3).

Today, however, when there is any form of untoward happening, such as the pandemic, there are stringent demands for rapid intervention and dynamic action. Then again, there are also people who do not want to do anything and loudly propagate their opinion in demonstrations and in the media. What position is the right one? Mencius continues,

There are few in the world who do not "help their sprouts grow." And there are those who do not "weed"—they have simply given the whole task up as useless. But the ones who tug on the sprouts to help the grow, they are worse than useless for they do harm! (Eno 2016, 40)

These two positions of strong interference and refusal to do anything are clearly present in the modern debate about the right to die. Some want to help life grow so much that they are tearing it to pieces, focusing on saving lives at all cost with no regard of the quality of life that remains. But what about being allowed to die? Can saving a life at any cost be a greater good than letting someone die with dignity? The life-prolonging measures of modern medicine no longer prolong life: they only delay death, as if they wanted to forbid dying

In the words of Mencius, such measures no longer help the grain but only destroy everything living that could one day become weeds. The same also applies to the lockdown during the pandemic with its harmful side effects on people's lives, which in turn is much like the use of pesticides in modern agriculture. A weed killer like glyphosate destroys all conceived as evil as well as what is really good. The environment is diminished, the living space of animals and plants is poisoned, and in the end human beings come to suffer. In this regard, too, Mencius has advice for the local ruler:

> If you regulate fishing nets so that fine-woven ones may not be used in the pools and ponds, there will be more fish than the people can eat. If you allow hatches and axes to be used in the woods only in proper season, there will be more lumber than the people can use. (1A3; Eno 2016, 19)

On the other hand, there are those "who do not weed," who think that all measures are superfluous because they believe nothing will happen and there is no point bothering. Such people need conspiracy theories to get their fears under control.

What, then, should one do in this situation? Obviously find some middle ground. Taiji and Qigong offer an exercise system of daily practice that allows people to increase their self-healing powers and maintain a calm composure in all kinds of circumstances. This causes the flood-like *qi* to move as intended and thereby strengthens the immune system, documented in numerous scientific studies. Restoring, elevating, and maintaining the flood-like *qi* is the best way to live life; it also forms an effective form of protection against disturbance and disease.

It is quite possible that Mencius himself practiced such exercises. As he says, this kind of *qi* is "generated through the long accumulation of righteous actions," which indicates firm and strong dedication to self-cultivation.

For us, this means that we have to keep at it constantly and practice daily. Such are the "righteous actions," the performance of duty, we have to dedicate ourselves to. And soon we come to feel good about it. We all know from experience that when we begin to practice out of a sense of duty, performing daily even when we do not feel like doing it, comfort and exhilaration follow. So, just start! Find serenity in these difficult times! And, of course, do not forget to get enough sleep! This is another feature Mencius praises.

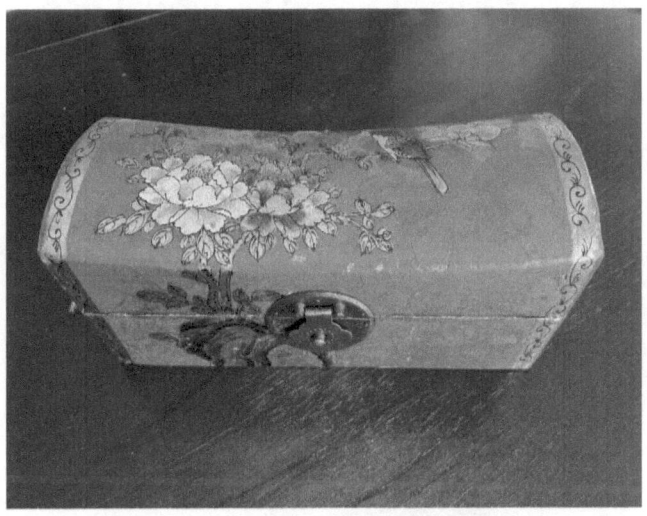

Fig. 63. Chinese Neck Support for Sleep.

10
Testimonials of Master-Disciples

Klaus Vorpahl, Taiji Master

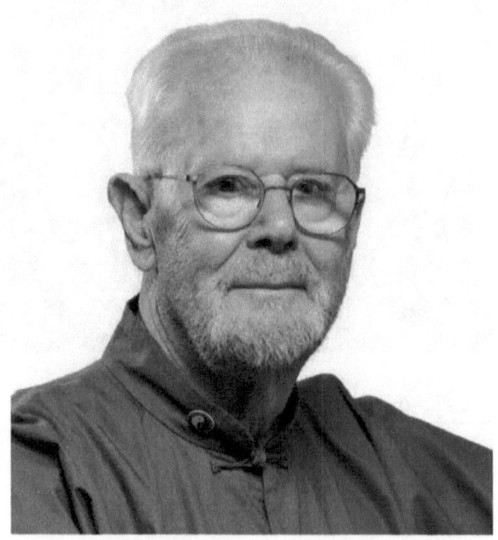

After nearly forty years of practice, I can no longer say what the benefits of Taiji are. Nor do I know what life is like without Taiji. On the walls of my studio, I only have a rubbing of the *Neijing tu* (Chart of Internal Passageways) from the White Cloud Monastery in Beijing, plus two pieces of calligraphy and a few small golden cardboard cards that say: "Practice—Practice—Practice." Practice never ends in Taiji. In the tradition of the Yang family, the form and the stages of concentration are only a prerequisite for practice, in order to eventually leave it behind and be able to return to the beginning.

A new beginning every day—what results from this can be called a rooted life. Finding yourself again and again in an area without results requires a certain perseverance. It is also important to keep clarifying what we are doing and with what ideas and goals we are doing what we are doing. The paths to be followed require the accompaniment of a master, a companion who knows the way. Those who have found it should not forget to bow in gratitude from time to time.

Dardo Lessmann, Taiji Master

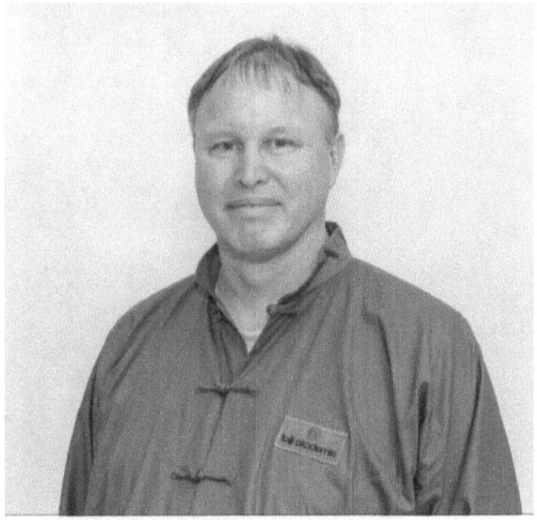

There is a Zen saying in Japanese that describes very nicely why I always leave class feeling so strengthened:

Mei reki reki -- Nothing is hidden,
Ro do do -- Everything is evident.

The first line presents the image of a drop of dew forming on a blade of grass, glistening in the morning sun. It arises from the meeting of the most diverse influences and is beautiful in its clarity and uniqueness. Such are the moments of realization that come up again and again in our joint work in the Taiji Academy, and which I can enjoy with a deep feeling of happy *qi*.

The second line describes a meadow in the morning sun, complete with innumerable many dewdrops, whose refreshing effect strengthens the heart and spirit. How nice to be able to enjoy them in their entirety!

This image always makes it clear to me how precious these moments are, when perception and consciousness are sharpened in the moment— and how infinitely numerous these moments are actually around us that just have to be discovered.

With this in mind, I am looking forward to a long beautiful journey of discovery to these moments that arise from our time together.

Sibel Cirsi

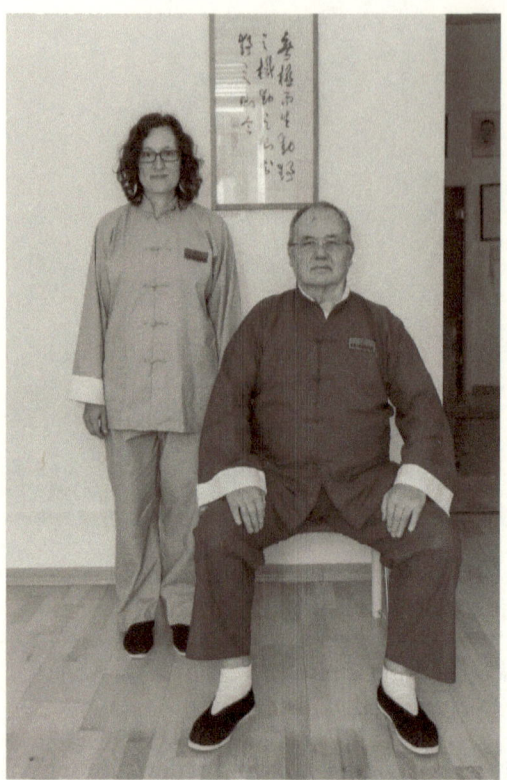

My first week-long experience of Frieder Anders's Taiji in Tuscany came exactly at the right time: I had been in doubt for quite a while whether Taiji was still the right path for me. I had the feeling that, while it was generally good for me and I had a lot of fun with it, there must be more to it than what I had been able to discover.

His first words after examining my form were: "You are already doing a lot of solar work." What that meant in detail was not clear to me at the time. Only much later I realized that my body was already trying to go in the direction that was right for me, which is why I had not been able to cope with some of the guidelines my other teachers offered and the practice had not felt good. Having never heard of the breathing types before, I spent most of my time in Tuscany becoming more familiar with doing Taiji as an exhaler. It was truly eye-opening. It felt good and I wanted to know more, learn more, and dig deeper.

In due course, I completed instructor training, but did not stop there: First I became a course instructor, then a teacher, and now I am a master-disciple. Frieder Anders has accompanied me on this path—as guide, helper me, supporter, and cheerleader. But he also challenged me, and he will continue to do so. When some move or form did not work right away, he made me understand it through other approaches. In the end, I am always rewarded by gaining another step on the way to championship. His excellent instruction on the different versions depending on the breathing type have encouraged me to continue on this path, to refine my feeling for my Taiji and now my passion to pass it on to anyone interested.

I hope I can continue to discover and learn lots of new things on this path and keep on teaching future students.

Manfred Bauer

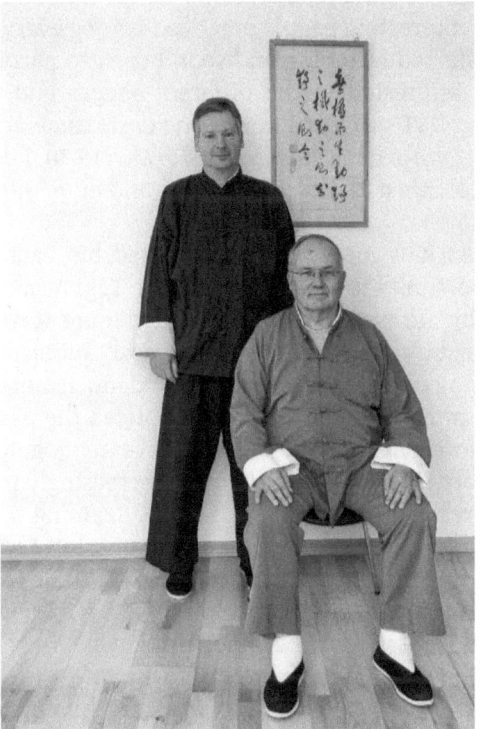

Discovering and practicing Taiji is an interesting and invigorating path. Yes, I think that describes it very well: we are on the right track. On a path full of interesting discoveries that always has an invigorating effect on me. For me, Taiji is a goal, one of the "Big Five for Life" as described in the book by John Strelecky, a pillar that stands at the core purpose of my existence. Just like my family (another of my "Big Five"), Taiji contributes significantly to my success in life as long as I practice and take care of it daily.

As a little boy I learned judo and also tried out ball sports. But my fascination was with the martial arts. I studied Judo, Jiu Jitsu, Karate, and a little

Aikido. I met many great teachers and masters who were always willing to teach me something new and quench my thirst for knowledge. I am deeply grateful to them all!

Early on, when I was still young, I discovered the positive effect different Qigong exercises had on my well-being. In my professional life, too, these exercises have proven to be ideal companions for my health. Because I travel a lot, I need to find local opportunities to train wherever I am. Qigong takes up so little space that there is always a place for it. A terrace or a meadow is sufficient.

In 1987, I started to look for more practitioners whenever I had the time, sometimes early in the morning, sometimes later in the day. And there they were. Whether in San Francisco, New Orleans, or on Lake Washington in Seattle, lots of interesting people practiced Qigong everywhere—but they also did Taiji! I started watching and soon began to participate. I became more and more interested in the different shapes and movements and bought books and DVDs to learn more. One day I came across Frieder Anders's book, *Das chinesische Schattenboxen: Tai Chi* (1979). I decided to go and see him. Ever since, my path has grown more and more interesting over the years.

A lot changed: kids got bigger, jobs changed, but Taiji stayed. In 2011, I first had the opportunity to take courses at the Taiji Academy in Frankfurt. I was fascinated by the aspects that were valued there. It was not only about the big yang form, but also about legs, arms, neck, spirals, correct standing, the holistic twisting of the body, breathing, and much more. There was a lot to discover, and practicing did me good! I noticed the positive changes in myself. My self-awareness increased, the movements guided by the spirit got more and more interesting and became increasingly meditative. It was the logical progression to attend the teacher training in 2013, then and spending many intensive hours with the grandmaster. I wish to thank him for patiently guiding me and always letting me try things out!

In May 2016, Frieder Anders appointed me a master-disciple. It is said that only the transmission of the inner principles of authentic Taiji preserves the teaching. It passes from master to disciple, who in due course becomes the master of the next generation. I found this entirely correct. Only in this way can I preserve the authentic tradition and continue to learn throughout my life. But it only represents one side. For Frieder Anders, Taiji is also a living legacy that breaks with tradition and continues to develop it further. I enjoy that this Taiji is not a rigid hierarchical structure to which one must submit in order to find one's own worth. Practicing according to breathing types has benefited me greatly. Thank you for this openness and the acceptance of change!

Practicing Taiji and Qigong, day after day, is always an interesting and invigorating experience! I'm enjoying it today, tomorrow, and the day after.

I always want to continue along this one interesting path. I look forward to every new step.

Brigitte Lagemann

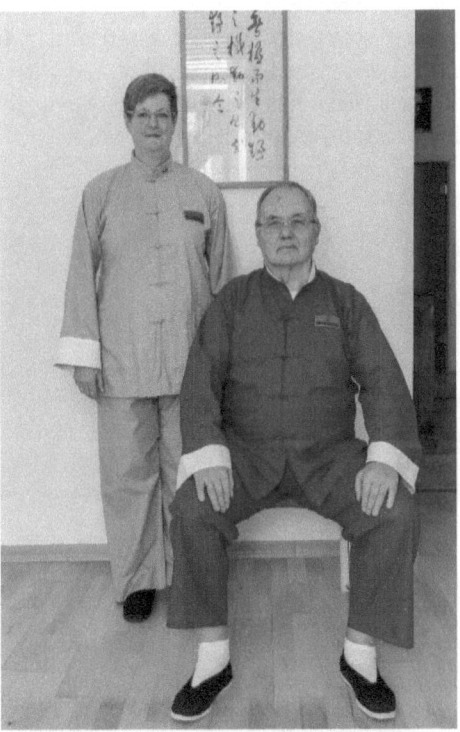

I was not even consciously looking for Taiji. I took an educational leave and studied Qigong, then decided to experiment with Taiji on the next. At that time, I got to know the beginning of the Taiji form in the Yang style. The movements were good for me, they were smooth, and I did not even have to overcome my weaker self. In a positive way, the practice was tiring, yet relaxing and calming at the same time.

As a result, I got curious and wanted to learn the entire form. I attended an open-door event at the Taiji Academy and got more input on breathing types. According to the test, I was a solar exhaler. I felt that working from this posture suited me very well. It was all natural. I did not have to relearn any-thing either.

I can imitate the movement sequences in the mode of a lunar inhaler and explain them to myself theoretically, but I do not have the same feelings about them. Rather, I find them rather uncomfortable.

When practicing, all my focus and concentration are directed inward. What are my muscles doing? Can I root myself well, ground myself, and let go at the same time? Taiji means a lot of body work and also a great deal of introspection. On the other hand, it also sharpens sensitivity to the outside world. It is always astonishing that the greatest power lies in doing nothing, in being light.

Taiji makes me more balanced, relaxed, and content; at the same time, gives me inner power, strength, and a soft sense of happiness that constantly resonates through my being. I take all of that with me into everyday life. The fascination with Taiji has not let go of me over the years. I still experience practicing as a journey of self-discovery.

Marion Hartung

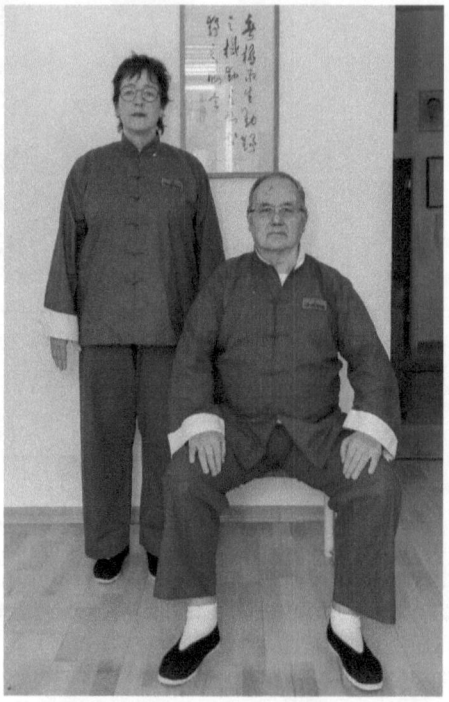

My path led me to Frieder Anders in 2008. I went together with my partner Andreas Korycik, who had been practicing Taiji in a club for many years. However, he did not make any progress there, unable to develop his full potential: the *qi* bubbled in him, but did not get into the flow.

For me, everything was still in the early stages. I had only noticed that nobody in my partner's club could show me the way. It was always just: "Feel inside yourself, and all will be fine . . ." I stood there alone and was allowed to spend hours stumbling around on the wrong track, because I did not even know what to feel.

At the Taiji Academy, on the other hand, everything suddenly became clear. I finally felt what I was doing and noticed the effects. I noticed how the flowing energy calmed my monkey mind and found a way for the *qi* to evolve.

My partner Andreas soon developed in huge steps. I followed him and Frieder Anders because I felt how invigorating the practice was, how it afforded me an inner peace and a strength that has influenced my life positively and powerfully to the point where I almost consider it a fountain of youth.

I especially like the weapon forms. The most valuable thing for a teacher is that you can regularly pass on your skills. Students' questions keep on showing me that I do not have all the answers or that I have to question myself again. In this way, my development is enormously promoted.

After almost thirteen years of Taiji, I have arrived in the inner circle of the master-disciples, even if this is only the beginning of a long path that will not end. I feel that thanks to Frieder Anders's decades of practice, we students make fewer detours and sometimes even take shortcuts that we would not have mastered without these decades of experience. I hope to be able to absorb this knowledge for many, many years to come.

Daniel Ackermann

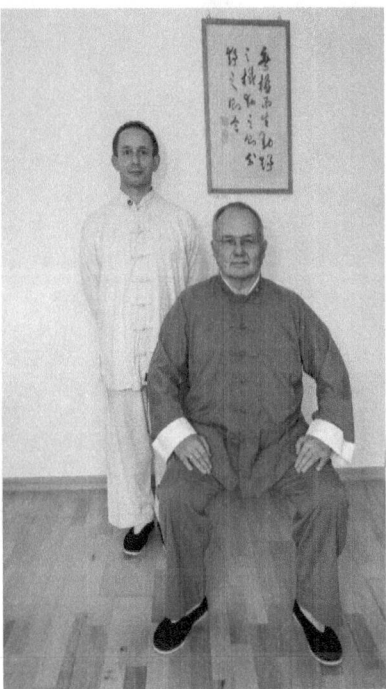

My first experience of Taiji was a form called Tai Chi Kineo. Lacking depth, it focused mainly on esoteric posturing. I quickly became dissatisfied, noting that there was no noticeable development. To this day, after more than twenty years of experience, I still use this example as a contrast to clarify the difference between external and internal forms of Taiji.

Internal Taiji is a great playing field for physical and mental development opportunities. Body and mind are constantly faced with new challenges and subjected to an ongoing growth process.

Everyone has potential, but it often gets stuck in us and, in the worst case, withers away. Inner Taiji is an excellent instrument not only to promote this potential, but also to carry it to the "outside." So-called *qi* tests and various partner exercises are more than helpful here. Cognitive dissonances are overcome and the feeling for one's own self is sharpened in exchange with exercise partners. Cultivating character leads to more social skills in dealing with each other.

Thomas Stroh

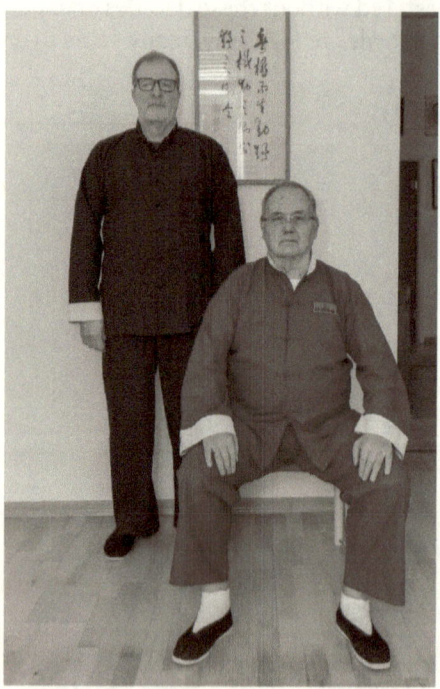

"What is Taiji? What can it do? It is not a dance, but a martial art, yet not aimed at developing muscle strength. Taiji is health practice, meditation in motion, the only self-defense method that uses the power of the mind alone to move the inner energies."

In 1982, while searching for a martial art that would be doable while getting older, I came across the passage cited above in an article about Taiji in the magazine *Warum*. The author was Frieder Anders. Since then, it has accompanied me with sometimes more and sometimes unfortunately less commitment. Nevertheless, the certainty remains that one can only improve and grow free from ideology or religion through constant practice. With the help of my great teacher, I continue to realize and perceive small advances on the path to inner power. Taiji is concentration, contemplation, mindfulness, and physical exercise coupled with the confidence of developing one's *qi*. The subtle examination of movement and breathing is what makes this art of movement so fascinating. I am deeply grateful for the long journey together with a true master.

Katja Möller

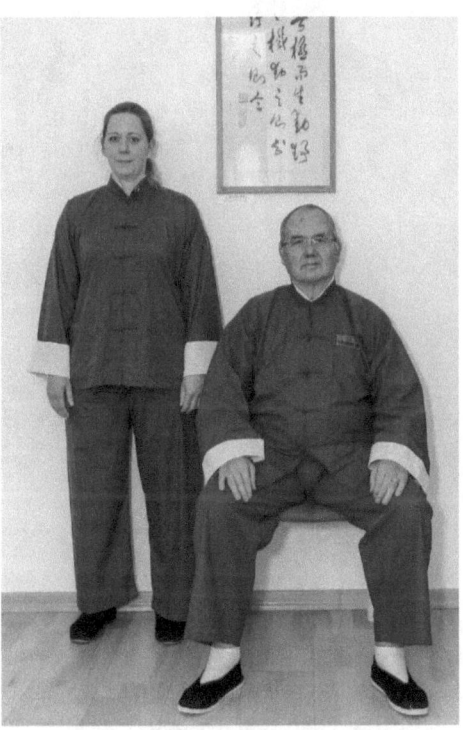

For me, inner power cannot be put into words: it has to be experienced. Maybe the best way to describe it is in the words of Zen Master Kinoshita: "playing along the path." Constant practice, quiet listening and feeling into your own body, muscular and mental letting go—those are essential.

In addition, there are practical tests with a partner and constant work with an experienced master, who guides the adept along the right path according to specific requirements—always there, always encouraging personal development. And in between there are situations of knowing that, according to Count Dürckheim, can be described as a "state of mind of enjoying the path" (1975, 60). Those brief times of full realization of lightness, of "acting in nonaction" keep me motivated to continue learning and playing.

Uwe Kroggel

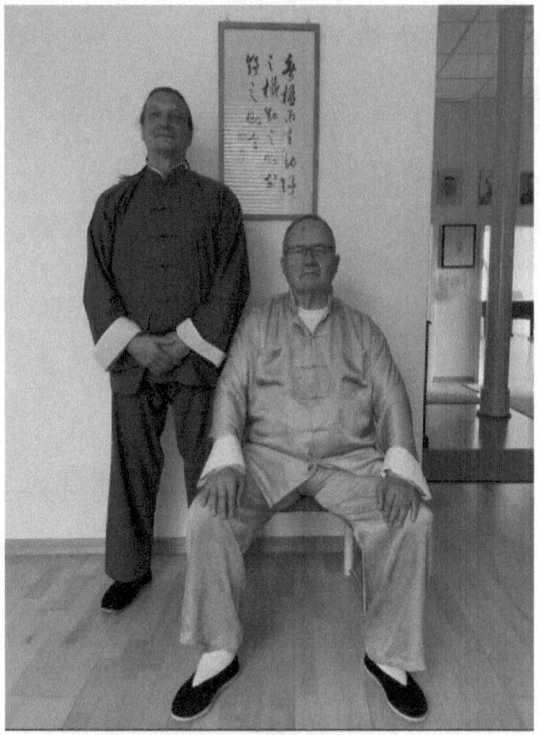

First of all, I have to perceive my body. When pressure or stress arise, I have to manage not to get tense, to release it again and again, but still be there. For me, it is important that I can feel my body, because only then can I also perceive the other person. I have to perceive the ground below, but also the sky above. I cannot put into words what happens next, I can only experience it myself. For me, inner power is satisfaction with oneself.

Rainer Weffer

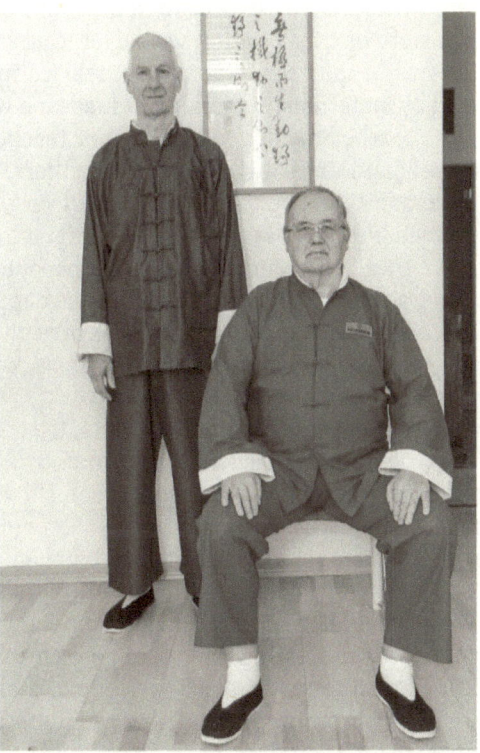

The inscription on the Apollo Temple in Delphi reads *gnothi seautón,* "know thyself." This has become my motto. Trying to understand myself, others, and the world almost automatically led me to meditation and Taiji. In my opinion, both are about the development of consciousness. While in meditation, I begin by paying attention to breathing, then observe thoughts and emotions, and eventually learn to accept them for the plain enjoyment of being. In Taiji, my focus is more on the joy of conscious movement in space and getting to know my body and spirit.

I first stated meditating by practicing Japanese Zen, later turned to Tibetan Dzogchen. Here, the term *tendrel* is central: it indicates an awareness that we do not exist as independent egos but are connected to everything. To put it bluntly, everything is connected to everything else.

This is exactly what fascinated me about Taiji, as I studied it first with Master Chu King-Hung, then—and to this day—with Frieder Anders. Everything is connected in the practice. The movement of the right arm generates more power when it is coordinated with the left and when head and feet are in the right position. Even the position of toes or fingers becomes conscious. Of course, breathing is central, especially when considering the breathing types, but even the mental attitude has an impact. For example, it makes a significant difference whether you expect something or not.

When I was in state of coordination with everything, on occasion—in moments when I hardly expected it—an almost magical power arose that cannot be explained by materialistic thinking. It made me want more of this other dimension and sparked my desire to become a teacher so that I could study more intensively and share my practice with others.

Over time, as an additional bonus, I experienced various health effects that I had not expected. Prone to depression and fatigue from an early age, I now no longer have these problems. Happy *qi* has become a regular experience. Just practicing a short form makes me alert and happy. With the help of Qigong exercises, also taught as part of the Taiji curriculum, I managed to control several severe allergies, asthma, and intense back pain due to herniated discs. Both my gait and my posture changed.

I also observed similar effects on my students, feeling both delighted and deeply grateful. Depressives became cheerful and relaxed; curmudgeons turned social and friendly. Many postural defects visibly improved. Plus, there was so much happy *qi*! Best of all, these outcomes did not depend on doing the exercises perfectly. It was enough to try them seriously. Those who simply came to class regularly and practiced, preferably without great expectations, were successful, regardless of age or previous knowledge.

I also experienced an interesting interaction with meditation. Long, often week-long sitting meditations regularly led to incredible experiences of the here and now, but my body did not cooperate and showed symptoms of illness. This reminds me of Bodhidharma, who observed something similar in his students and therefore taught them additional martial exercises in his residence at the Shaolin Monastery. Using Taiji in a similar manner, it became a supplement to meditation and more. When I meditate, conscious movement becomes easier. When I practice Taiji and Qigong, I am more alert while meditating and stay healthy.

In conclusion, I can say that the movements of Taiji, standing Qigong, and sitting meditation fulfill are my dream team of self-cultivation, a multiple win-win-win story.

Part Two

Fundamental Concepts

11
Basic Principles

Dao

> Don't intervene, and there is nothing that is not done.
> —*Daodejing* 37

Dao, literally the "way," describes how something runs optimally. Originally the term was not only used by Daoists but by the ancient Chinese elite to communicate excellence in general. Those who moved in Dao were superior in their behavior to others (Moeller 2001, 31-32).

Dao designates a path with a special interweaving of being and nonbeing, fullness and emptiness, presence and absence. It most closely corresponds to what psychologists call the "flow experience." After much training, practitioners get to a point where they no longer consciously perceive their activity. The difficult and laborious becomes easy: it happens as if of itself and flows naturally. The same thing happens during long-distance running: the longer you run, the more likely you can run almost effortlessly and no longer notice the effort.

In such an experience one enters what Daoists describe as the process of being in Dao. On the one hand, the ego of the runner disappears and becomes empty; on the other hand, the optimal way of running emerges. Without emptiness, there can be no perfection or effortless endurance. Fullness and emptiness are mutually interdependent, because only the absence of the ego allows the full presence of running. When the ego becomes conscious again, this disrupts the flow, and the trek becomes once again difficult and exhausting. In other words, Dao is present when fullness and emptiness are in balance.

Daoists have many images that illustrate this principle of interlocking fullness and emptiness: the valley, the bellows, the empty vessel, the doorway, and the wheel. They are all metaphors that show how something works through the combination of fullness and emptiness. The valley generates life without consuming itself; the bellows gives energy when it empties and refills. The empty vessel and the doorway are examples of a receiving space, an emptiness that fills the inside of a frame. The wheel, finally, shows how movement occurs on the basis of a connection of spokes to axle. Whether valley or bellows, vessel or doorway, or even wheel—they are all empty in the center, and only this nonbeing, emptiness, or hollowness makes it possible for them to fulfill their purpose. What can optimally fulfill its purpose is in Dao.

In the West, Dao has often been misunderstood as something metaphysical, a kind of unmoving mover that keeps the world going. But the Chinese worldview is more concrete: The best strategy or best user's instructions, the most effective order for optimal effectiveness is Dao. Accordingly, there are many Daos: Dao of heaven, Dao of earth, Dao of humanity, but also Dao of domination or of warfare. Dao is "a kind of way of all ways, a method of all methods, a pattern of all patterns" (Moeller 2001, 30). Whoever moves in Dao is a sage, a person who, according to Zhuangzi, is subject to external change without ever changing within. Taiji is a way of attaining Dao.

There are two main lines of Daoist wisdom, religious and philosophical. The goal of both is immortality. Followers of religious Daoism strive to transform the body into a kind of *perpetuum mobile*, a wheel that keeps running indefinitely. This vision gave rise to physical exercises, nutritional teachings, and spiritual practices that serve to maintain health and are intended to guarantee an almost infinitely long life. This is how Taiji and Qigong came about.

Philosophical Daoists work with meditation and the study of texts, hoping to attain a state of consciousness that accepts the cycle of life and death. People become immortal in spirit when death no longer bothers them. They attain nonattachment and serenity with the realization that they are a part of greater cosmos, which in essence consists of the constant alternation of life and death. The world to them is living movement—Dao.

The legacy of both, the intentional care for a healthy body and the vigorous pursuit of true serenity, is more relevant than ever in our hectic and unhealthy world today.

Probably in the 14th century, a martial art arose with the aim of developing inner power through the interaction of *qi* with consciousness, a way of letting an attacker bounce off without injury. The legendary founder of this martial art was Zhang Sanfeng, a master of the external martial arts. At the age of seventy, he retired to Mount Wudang to seek wisdom and, according to legend, was inspired to create the internal martial art of Taiji while watching a snake fight a crane.

The original purpose of Asian martial arts was to learn to fight so one would not have to fight. This is where both, internal martial arts like Taiji and external ones like Gongfu, differ fundamentally from the Western idea of combat sports. Combat sports are about fighting, while martial arts are about refining and cultivating the body and the person as a whole.

External martial arts and combat sports train the body as a weapon. Eyes, fists, and feet learn to react quickly and fight effectively. The force used is external. Mass, weight, and muscle tension create momentum and strength, but not internal energy. Internal Taiji, on the other hand, develops inner power that works without muscular strength.

The two can be distinguished easily by looking at the type of movement: external martial arts are agile and intense, sometimes almost acrobatic; in internal martial arts one hardly moves, head and torso stay upright almost all the time. The lack of mobility is an advantage. External techniques get harder and more demanding with age, because they take a lot of strength and wear out the body. The reservoir of inner power, on the other hand, potentially continues to grow with age. This energy is optimally used in internal Taiji and only consumed minimally.

The 19th century was the heyday of this practice in China. At the time, it is said, no representative of an external martial art could ever defeat a Taiji master. The effectiveness of Taiji as a martial art is that the body becomes strong and elastic like a ball. After a while, the arms look like iron bars wrapped in cotton. They are only moved lightly and relaxed, but develop great strength and resilience. On the other hand, counter-rotating spiral movements of the head, spine, core, and legs are used but almost invisible. The body becomes a large ball with rotating, interlocking segments that deflect each attack like a ball thrown into the roulette wheel.

Spiraling Energy

Whoever follows Dao overcomes the limitations of ego-centered volition and integrates with the movements of the cosmos. Taiji does not regard the body merely as a physical entity but sees it essentially as consisting of energetic processes. With the right posture and movement, this microcosmic body becomes a harmonious part of the macrocosm. In both dimensions of the cosmos, energy moves in spirals and waves.

Spiraling fog, swirling clouds, whirlpools—the entire world consists of nothing but spirals, both on earth and in the greater universe. Even the human body is full of spiral structures—from the DNA double helix through the umbilical cord to the muscles of the heart and limbs. In nature they appear in climbing ivy, mussels and snails, as well as antlers, horns, and claws. Even in everyday life, things that are supposed to have a lot of power, such as a screw or a corkscrew, have a spiral shape.

Internal Taiji integrates the movements of the body into this ubiquitous interplay of spirals. Little by little, practitioners learn to develop their physical movement patterns into spirals. The energy this accrues is potentially infinite, because it is not trapped within the confines of the body. It affords a power that is not a mere mechanical force described according to the rules of solid-state physics.

The spirals of energy that go through the body in internal Taiji end in nothing—that is, they swing outward. Using internal energy means to start any movement as if it had already begun and never ending it with an abrupt stop. It is quite like a symphony concert. All the instruments move together and come to a clear stop at a certain moment, just as the conductor lowers his baton. At the same time, however, the music does not stop immediately, but continues to vibrate, then gently fades away. In the same way, movements in Taiji reach beyond the end and are carried out as if part of an endlessly turning wheel.

The wheel in Daoism and Taiji is a model of how movements run optimally. In the center of the wheel is the axle, the empty hub, with four distinct properties: it is central, empty, at rest, and unified.

Just as the hub is the center that enables the use of the wheel, every movement in Taiji needs a core in order to be able to work. Just as in a wheel, the axle, spokes, and rim are grouped around the center, which in itself is empty and consists of only an opening, so in Taiji, movements of arms, legs, and head revolve around the core. Just as a wheel only runs true when this empty center is at rest and remains immobile, lest it break, so in Taiji, one becomes unbalanced when the axis of the body slants. Just as in a wheel, the empty center holds the many parts together and combines them into a functioning unit, so in Taiji, the hands, feet, and torso move as if around a stationary, unchangeable core, the axis that connects heaven and earth.

Daoists also used the wheel as a model for the successful construction of any mechanism or organization, whether naturally grown or artificially constructed. In the state, the emperor was regarded as the core that remained idle and did not act, while officials and the people moved around him. This inactive center made it possible for the state come together as an optimally functioning whole. In the human body, the heart fulfills the same role: it is the pulsating but inherently immobile center, around which blood and all the other bodily functions circulate. The fundamental vision of Taiji as a return to natural patterns is fully realized when the body learns to move once more like a wheel.

Internal Taiji developed primarily in the image of the wheel, following Daoist ideas that claimed the body should move in this fashion. Here the core is in the lower abdomen, just below the navel, the center of gravity and the ocean of the *qi*. The body revolves around this immobile core in all its movements. Because it remains empty and does not move, the arms and legs, like spokes of a wheel, do nothing of themselves, but are moved by the core. In this manner, the body reaches the fullness of internal energy.

The back remains stretched during all movements and only inclines along one axis with the entire trunk. Arms and legs become round again and again as they move, as if they forming a wheel or holding a ball. The upright torso and the rounded shape of arms and legs open the joints and expand the breathing space. This creates the so-called flow of *qi*: a flow of energy through the entire body.

This flow, then, can be guided in a circular path through the torso, using specific breathing techniques. This creates an internal wheel, in due course followed by the movements of arms and legs. The spiraling motion of the limbs mimics the rolling back and forth of a wheel, in due course coordinated with the breath and the circular flow of internal energy. Years of practice lead to a flow experience of great power and lightness. As the Chinese proverb says, over time the practitioner becomes "flexible like a child, healthy like a lumberjack, and calm like a sage."

Yin and Yang

Internal energy works through an alternation of fullness and emptiness, and allows the adept to defeats the opponent in nonaction. His power bounces, off because he cannot find an empty spot to penetrate. Such energy develops from movements, in which fullness and emptiness constantly alternate and interact.

The Chinese describe this in terms of yin and yang, which also denote the pattern of the world in general: life and death, day and night, male and female, inhaling and exhaling, up and down, and so on—all these phenomena match the concepts of fullness and emptiness.

Internal Taiji has an advanced level, the so-called Yin-Yang Form. It divides the predetermined, constant sequence of movements into yin and yang phases. In the yin phases, the body withdraws, arms lower or close and move down toward earth. In the yang phases, the body advances, arms rise or open and reach for the sky. Yin phases are considered empty because they absorb energy from heaven or the sky and transmit it to earth. The same thing happens with the attacker's energy. Yang phases are considered full because they are filled with ascending earth energy and release this energy into vastness.

In the Taiji solo form, a yin phase always alternates with a yang phase. While these are dry runs that actually relate to an opponent, they are performed without a partner. Only in push-hands exercises with a partner can the alternation of fullness and emptiness be tested physically.

The point of push-hands is to experience how the yin and yang movements complement each other in every moment and turn into their opposite at the end of each phase. Alertness and sensitivity are more important than the use of muscular strength.

Partners face each other and keep one or both arms in constant light contact. In a fixed sequence of forward and backward rolling movements, the goal is to throw your partner off balance while not losing your own. They each tries to keep their footing safe and only go back and forth as far as they can without endangering their center. A full yang movement advancing is followed by an empty yin movement withdrawing. One partner's yang movement is the other's yin. Together they form a whole of yin and yang, as depicted in the Taiji symbol.

Force in Taiji must never be met with the same opposing force. A yang movement that pushes forward should not be countered with a yang movement of the partner, otherwise pressure merely responds to counter pressure: the martial art becomes external. The goal is to neutralize the yang force with a yin movement. The attacker's power is dissipated into the ground and exhausted without an actual hit. Once the force is neutralized, the other partner begins a yang movement.

If both partners remain well centered, the mechanics of a gear train that constantly rolls back and forth is created. As soon as one of the two partners falls forward into a void or stumbles backward, he has lost his central axis, seduced by the other's movements. Maybe he took his yang movement too far forward and lost his centeredness as a result; quite possibly was too lax when backing away; or, again, he used muscle strength to block the yang energy so that it could be dissipated and threw him back.

The decisive factor with visible success is that whoever falls has only themselves to blame. Taiji uses power without harshness: no one intends to trip the other or use rough pulls and shoves. The partner should fall of his own accord, out of his own weakness, because he was greedy and maneuvered himself into a bad position. Of course, the victorious partner lures him into this weak position and provokes the weakness that he can exploit, but nobody forces the loser with insidious tricks or hidden violence.

Push-hands exercises are by no means a powerless and harmony-seeking stirring of the arms back and forth that blurs all opposites. They are a vivid and vibrant experience of the dynamics of yin and yang.

Harmony of yin and yang arises as a result of the struggle between the two forces and not due to some kind of esoteric, primordial condition. To unfold the power in both directions, the alternation of fullness and emptiness must be clearly separated, mentally and physically. If any change causes an external effect, this is the necessary consequence of the interaction of one's inner power and the other's weakness. This matches traditional Chinese military strategy, which too is based primarily on exploiting the other's weaknesses as effortlessly as possible.

As one becomes more skillful, the movements in push-hands become increasingly smaller until only sparks of large circular patterns are needed to uproot the other. The yin movement can be so small that you hardly see it, but it acts like a trapdoor, giving the opponent the feeling of falling into an abyss. The body reacts involuntarily with a shock that blocks its actions and the flow of energy. Once empty, a simple yin twist can unbalance the other completely, then lift him off his feet with a yang movement.

In this uprooting, when the trapdoor opens, the partner is full of false fullness—tension and sluggish power. Twisted out of proportion, he loses his centeredness and his standing without even being aware of this. He does not understand why he was uprooted. With perfect technique—when all spirals interact with the breath in a certain way—the effect is enormous: as soon as contact occurs, internal energy rotates and pushes the attacker back. This happens so fast that it is actually like bouncing off. Whoever masters the techniques of inner power defeats his opponent without fighting.

Nonaction

The concept of nonaction (*wuwei*) occupies a central place in Daoism and it is also the essence of internal Taiji. The full expression is "acting through nonaction" (*wei wuwei*). The basic idea is simple: if you are in harmony with Dao, you don't have to do anything and things unfold of themselves.

This not acting can be understood in very different ways. The Seven Sages of the Bamboo Grove, for example, a group of eccentric 3rd-century poets practiced it by retiring from their positions as government officials and living in solitude in the countryside. They did not act on behalf of society and were even respected for it!

Of course, nonaction in Taiji is not like this. Rather, it means four things. First, it signals an emptiness that allows the growth of inner power; second, it means not interfering with the spontaneous running of the body wheel; third it connotes waiting for a strategic weakness in the opponent; and fourth, it indicates having an open heart and an empty mind.

The Daoist concept of nonbeing (*wu*) indicates emptiness and the absence or openness of things that manifest in a certain way. For example, a valley or a bellows function because of the empty space the afford, because of what is not there. This is the opposite of the concept of fullness and presence, that is, of being (*you*). For example, the mountain that matches the valley is *you*. It is a core facet of Daoist thought that everything that is full and present can only arise from emptiness and nonbeing. The *Daodejing* says, "All things in the world come from being. And being comes from nonbeing" (ch. 40).

In a bellows, wind—that is, inner power—only arises from the emptiness of the device as it is set in motion. Taiji practitioners must be empty of volition and emotion, both toward themselves and their opponents. They must not even want to grow inner power for themselves. The only thing they have to do is decide on a certain movement, then do nothing but that movement: this is where inner power arises.

If you do something without doing anything, you set in motion a spontaneous process. In Taiji and Qigong this means that, through the body movements, *qi* circulates around the empty core. The movements are an end in themselves in their execution: they do not follow a particular intention or volition. Action happens without the intellect intervening. Inner power appears almost coincidentally—it is not desired or planned or created. It arises spontaneously: now movements at one with Dao.

This ideal is expressed particular with the three words *yi*, *qi*, and *jin*—intention, energy, and power. As Mencius says, "Where the intention goes, the *qi* follows." This is how inner power arises. A mind filled with direction or desire automatically directs attention and intention to something and causes all movements to follow. In everyday life, this means you can take a glass off the table or put it back again.

Something similar happens in Taiji, only with highly conscious attention. For this, the mind must learn to wait. First, we empty it of all stress, urgency, and anger; then we focus intention and carry out whatever movement the mind has chosen without any ulterior motive. A troubled heart or restless mind cannot wait: it wastes the movement, letting inner power arise only accidentally. Causing an opponent to fall is the result of a correct and conscientious movement sequence but it happens with an easy intention, without actively wanting it. This also holds true for military strategy:

> A Chinese general makes no conjectures, elaborates no arguments, constructs nothing. He set up no hypotheses, makes not attempt to calculate what is probable. On the contrary, all his skill lies in the earliest possible detection of the slightest tendencies that may develop....
>
> The whole of military strategy, when confronting an enemy, could even be summed up by the following double maneuver: never present the slightest crack to the enemy so that he can never get a hold on you and will be bound to slide about with no means of penetrating your facade; at the same time, watch for the development on his side of the slightest crack: progressively widening into a breach, it will eventually make it possible to attack him without risk. (Jullien 2004, 68-70)

This is an excellent description of the right strategy in Taiji. It is not about being able to attack the opponent at any time with the most sophisticated methods possible. On the contrary: the use of internal energy is only worthwhile if and when the opponent shows a crack or becomes brittle. Weak spots are areas of nonbeing that can be easily and effortlessly pierced to gain victory with little effort.

At the highest level of mastery, a wise Taiji master can find such weak points at any moment. More inexperienced adepts, on the other hand, first have to develop a yet different ability in push-hands or when dealing with opponents: they have to learn to wait and do nothing. If no crack appears and the opponent seems untouchable, they must not attack. According to both Chinese strategy and Taiji principles, this would only exhaust power unnecessarily. Still, a good strategist does not remain idle while waiting; rather, he nurtures his power to the greatest possible level.

For Daoists, the spiritual center of the person is not in the head but in the heart. According to Taiji principles, the heart and mind should be empty and do nothing during practice. Emptiness here means being free from all volition and emotions. An empty heart-mind directs the attention and thus the energy entirely to the movement and its course. Pure energy, unclouded by the urge to achieve something, remains free from fear or aggression.

An empty heart means being free from emotions and passions in one's action. No anger, hatred, fear, or deviousness, but also no desire for devotion and harmony must guide one's actions if inner power is to grow. This may sound ethical, but it is really quite the opposite: Daoists tend to ridicule Confucians for the rigidity of their moral rules. In fact, it is mainly about strategy: defense and resilience are greater when emotions do not disturb mental clarity. Only with an empty heart will one not suffer unnecessary hurt by the attacker and live to be victorious.

An empty heart is free from anger and aggression, but not so empty that it goes limp and does not want anything anymore. Withdrawal and surrender are not a virtue, as some Taiji practitioners have suggested. They are the ones who buckle down limply at any attack and fail to maintain their own space. The mind collapses, and the body wheel turns into a figure of eight.

A focused yet empty heart that can wait, one that neither gives way nor resists, leads movements in Dao and penetrates the opponent's cracks.

Body Posture

Traditional Chinese cosmology posits three basic powers: heaven, earth and humanity. All three form one integrated unit, with humanity linking the other two, mediating between the power above and that below. This means that the human task is clear: people should attain their true inner power by uniting heaven and earth within themselves.

For Taiji, this means that all life takes place in a field of tension between gravity—the yin of earth—and reach—the yang of heaven or the sky. Proper posture, therefore, balances and connects the two. The knees are slightly bent so that the center of gravity sinks closer to the ground. The core in the lower abdomen connects to gravity, while head, torso, and spine lift upward as if sitting upright. The crown grows upward. In this way, both poles are perfectly balanced and united. In this posture, which always remains straight, the body moves slowly, gliding and flowing so as never to lose the connection between heaven and earth.

This posture represents and preserves nothing less than the world order of ancient Chinese thought. Under the Tang dynasty (688-907), even headstands were prohibited so that people would not "turn the world order upside down." In Taiji, uprightness is never lost: there are no leaps (at least not in Yang style), no falls, and no acrobatic moves that bend the body and disrupt its straight line.

This relaxed yet tight, upright, and unbent posture in Taiji allows the person to absorb and release power. It corresponds to way of being that the

Israeli physicist and movement teacher Moshe Feldenkrais calls "tonic adjustment," from the Greek word *tonos*, which signifies the tension of a string on an instrument. Without muscle contraction, it maintains uprightness in the push-pull of heaven and earth.

Taiji adepts stand firmly on the ground and use gravity optimally, so they neither overcome it nor surrender to it. In contrast, Western competitive sports follow the motto "higher, faster, further." Its proponents want to lift off from the earth and become weightless, just like classical ballet dancers rise in graceful jumps. Practitioners of other movement arts like Yoga tend to stick more closely to the ground as they enter poses that the body could never perform standing up: in many ways they are too heavy. Internal Taiji seeks the right level of heaviness and insists on standing firmly on the ground. It creates lightness, stability, and strength without tension.

Here the posture is like that of a small child who has just learned to walk. The knees are slightly bent and the body rocks from one foot to the other, creating a single line of gravity on the loaded leg. The torso remains stretched, the head is up, neither falling forward nor back, and the arms float and rotate with the movements of the body. The child optimally transmits the energy impulse that goes up from the feet and can easily jump up and down like a ball without any hindrance. Nothing stops the child's desire to move, no tension and no false slackness.

This kind of relaxed movement is much more difficult for adults. Even the normal upright posture with straight legs does not have a clear line of gravity. The straight walk dissipates the energy rising from the ground and puts unfavorable stress on the joints and spine. In external martial arts such as Karate or Gongfu, adepts dig into the ground or push themselves away from it, using muscular strength. They do not use the momentum that comes off the ground like a ball or a toddler.

Taiji students learn to absorb the energy that comes from the ground as an upward impulse and transform it with the breath into circular waves that spread throughout the body and can be used to grow inner power. Young children's grip is firm but not hard: they use inner power, not muscular strength. In order to recover this kind of power, people must learn to put themselves back into the correct relationship with gravity. Then it will revitalize rather than hinder or depress.

In order to connect with gravity, in Taiji, the body needs to sink. This sinking does not mean to go as low to the ground as possible and contract all the muscles in the leg. On the contrary: sinking happens through relaxation. Only a tonic, upright body without muscle tension can collect the *qi* in the lower elixir field and let it circulate freely through the meridians. Sinking is an active-passive act that consists of letting go. The body will naturally straighten when one lets go of weight and allows it to slide into the floor: it is not something we do but a gift we receive. No intentional wanting or acting must disturb the process once initiated: it must unfold on its own.

With a tensely upright body, as if standing at attention, *qi* cannot sink down and gets stuck above. The center shifts from the lower abdomen to the chest, and the Ocean of *Qi* below the navel is cut off. Collecting *qi* in the lower abdomen is essential for developing a self-awareness that rests in itself and comes from the core. This allows serenity to grow and forms the foundation of a vital organism. In contrast to Westerners who tend to exaggerate standing stiffly at attention and have the urge to be active, the Chinese emphasize the opposite: they often let their chest sag in such a way that they block the *qi* in the lower abdomen. This posture, which creates an artificial immobilization, unfortunately is standard in many Taiji styles that are too soft and forgiving.

With correct body tension, *qi* sinks down and moves along a consciously controlled circuit throughout the body: up the back and down the front, into the lower abdomen.

In Taiji, the optimal posture is often described in terms of rooting, indicating a position that is so secure no attacker can knock one over. Adepts stand firmly, rooted in the ground like a plant. To do so, they shift their core down and get the feet to make secure contact with the earth. Gravity focuses where the body axis directs the weight into the ground. Someone standing centered in the chest does not have this quality of rooting and can easily be knocked over.

This technique is not about making oneself heavier than one actually is. A plant rooted deep grows skyward and always corrects toward moving vertically—like a tumbling doll. Because its center of gravity is so low, it cannot be knocked over and always straightens itself. In this sense, being rooted in Taiji is the foundation for straightening the body, but also for all upward-directed movements.

Body Movements

Taiji acknowledges five directions of moving the body in space: forward, backward, left turning, right turning, and—as a special case—calm and centered standing.

All these movements come from by the core, at the level of the navel. A shift of the core toward one leg, such as the front knee or the back foot, creates a connection between torso and ground: an axis to hold the weight. To center the weight clearly on this one (and only) body axis, the navel rotates almost imperceptibly in the direction of the desired line, not taking the pelvis or shoulders along. Without this one body axis, inner power cannot develop, because the *qi* rotating around enables free mobility with secure footing in all directions. As Moshe Feldenkrais says,

> Human beings are so highly developed in rotation that they can turn faster than most animals: in boxing, bullfighting, the Japanese martial arts, and

more . . . a collision with the charging attacker can be avoided by a mere sideways turn. The system is so well designed and mostly works so fast that self-preservation seems like a miracle. (1987, 183)

Going forward in Taiji, we shift the body weight from one leg to the other, quite similar to everyday walking. But there is an important difference. In everyday walking, we simply push the body mass back and forth; in Taiji, we shift the core, usually in an oblique direction.

The core moves from one foot to the other, and the torso involuntarily moves with it. This creates a slightly oblique movement toward the periphery, matching the direct path between the feet, where the body axis shifts. The center of gravity moves and is rooted in the new position. Only when the core has arrived, can the body settle: the weight follows the core, and *qi* can rise up. Inner power grows only from this posture, in close connection to heaven and earth. Internal *qi* peaks at the end of a movement, when it is briefly and imperceptibly stopped. Whenever the body settles on one foot through a core movement, internal energy spirals most strongly.

If Taiji practitioners want to move someone standing before them by activating inner power, they do not use body mass to push. Rather—invisible to the other—they pursue a diagonal track past him. They shift the core at an angle while their arms come straight at the opponent. If the arms are flexible at this point, that is, without intentional tension, the opponent cannot feel that something is coming toward him. He only notices the effect of inner power at the end of the movement force, when he finds himself uprooted.

Going backward, i. e., yielding to a force, occurs in the same manner. It happens never straight but is always diagonal or at an angle, a feature that serves to take the body out of the direct line of fire and reaches a strong position on the back leg. This oblique movement fools the opponent into thinking that it is straight. He cannot see the path of the core from the outside, and his power is drained.

If martial artists want to bring down an opponent, they use various techniques such as pushing, pulling, or throwing. Taiji balances these and makes sure one never falls. Whether push or pull, adepts neutralize them all by staying upright in a relaxed way, shifting the weight, and engaging in circular movements, thereby allowing the attack to come to nothing. Even if they get caught and uprooted, they will not fall but defuse the energy of the attack by performing small, elastic hops, sort of like a sparrow. By hopping backward, even if uprooted they can maintain their upright posture, connecting heaven and earth. This allows them to stick to the opponent without actually being in the prone position of defeat. There is no falling in Taiji.

According to Feldenkrais, falling constitutes a primal human fear. Other martial arts counter this by teaching ways to fall without injury.

Adepts of internal Taiji do not do so, but offer techniques to bring the opponent to the ground. Yet, they do not force him to fall with the painful application of muscular strength or body weight. Rather, they apply Taiji methods that serve to let the opponent fall by himself. Through the correct use of intention, energy, and power in conjunction with the internal spirals, they destabilize the opponent's body, and he loses his balance. Even when he is down, adepts do not apply mechanical blocks such as twisting the joints to the point where pain forces the attacker to surrender. Rather, they block his internal energy: he is surprised and upset finding himself suddenly on the ground without knowing how he got there. There is no fixed outcome to this situation; rather, the teaching is to parry and not attack.

If the opponent uses brute force and launches a throw, Taiji adepts defend themselves with inner power generated by the upright posture that connects heaven and earth. The opponent can no longer execute a throw because they are too stable. They give way at any body part where the opponent has them in a firm grip, leaving these sections to the opponent in order to recover uprightness and focus on rooting. This does not happen as a physical reflex through the voluntary tensing of muscles, which represent a rather rough effort that is usually weaker than the opposing force, combined as it is with throwing techniques. Rather, this recovery is guided from within, through the imagination. It extends beyond the limits of the body to potential infinity, and happens not through the contraction of the body but by intensifying the inherently dynamic posture brought about by the imagination. When the spirit guides, one can stand like a tree.

12

Inner Power

Yi and *Jin*

> The soft overcomes the hard.
> —Daodejing 37

Inner power can only be fully understood beyond the dualism of body and mind. The dualistic view that human beings consist of two very different substances, a mechanical body and a non-mechanical mind, goes back to the philosopher René Descartes. In the West, it still determines how people use their bodies: the mind should master the body, and all strength is just mechanical, the raw force of muscles. In China, this dualism never existed: mind and body are seen as two poles of a unit that can affect each other.

Here, as formulated in Daoism, human beings, as much as all living things, consist of "three treasures" (*sanbao*): life energy (*qi*), primordial essence (*jing*), and spirit (*shen*). They are located in the lower abdomen (*jing*), at the level of the solar plexus (*qi*), and in the head (*shen*). Spirit is evident in a person's bright eyes; it is the driving force of personality, yet it is just as physical as the other two. All three are located in the body, in energy repositories, known as elixir fields. In Taiji, all movements originate from the lower field; then spirit guides them toward the upper field, so that the life energy in the middle field can flow well and develop significant power.

Based on this vision, most vibrantly activated in internal alchemy, the physical culture in ancient China was quite different from that of competitive sports as it developed in Europe. Taiji and Qigong emerged from the meditation exercises of Daoists, Buddhists, and shamans who wanted to establish a connection between the physical and spiritual realms. The body was to be spiritually infused and guided in specific directions, which according to religious Daoism were inhabited by gods and spirits (also called *shen*). Taiji and Qigong are essentially meditation for cultivating the three treasures rather than physical exercises in the Western sense.

The ability of the mind to guide the body is called *yi* in Chinese. *Yi* denotes mental activity—attention, ideas, thoughts, intention—and in Taiji means the ability of mental control or spiritual guidance. Attention precedes movement and *qi*. *Yi* senses and empathizes with physical and the mechanical processes: it anticipates movements in the mind before executing them.

The guiding spirit, however, is not the same as will and intention. In a way, *yi* also follows the body and is not just its leader. That is to say, after attention has grasped the object in the imagination, it waits for the impulse that marks the arrival of physical energy before it does anything. It cannot just do as it pleases, but is part of a team. This impulse, moreover, is so subtle that people tend not to notice it in everyday life.

Matching Chinese concepts, Volkmar Glaser created a neurophysiological model together with a holistic, psychosomatically oriented therapy he calls psychotonics. Building on the course of *qi* flowing through the meridians as defined in Chinese medicine, he developed basic forms of posture and movement that represent development stages of people in their attitude to the world. The attitude he calls "integral" realizes a state of *eutony*—a good tension in relation to the world. This is similar to the basic position of authentic Yang-style practice. According to Glaser, this integral attitude consists of what he calls trans-sensing, a feeling beyond self and body, in conjunction with an intention that wants to realize a project in the world (Grossmann-Schnyder and Glaser 1998).

Yi, the conscious spirit that guides the body in Taiji, has the characteristics of both trans-sensing and intentionality. It is actively geared toward moving and effecting something, yet and at the same time it seems to reside beyond the limits of the body. In everyday life, we constantly use *yi* without realizing it. When we pick up a cup, *yi* anticipates the movement, leading and directing it—there is automated, robotic grabbing. Even when jumping over a stream, *yi* reaches out to the other bank and guides the body to carry out the movement without hesitation. Intention and trans-sensing are both involved, and there is no voluntary or deliberate muscle contraction.

When *yi* is present, the mind is awake and empty. Its only job is to be with or ahead of the movements. It is calm and patient, free from emotions, and the movements it directs are slow and steady—all of equal importance. The mind reacts spontaneously and resolutely directs the movements, internalized after long practice to such a point that a reaction to any attack is automatic.

It always starts from the empty core, like the bear in the story "The Puppet Theater" by the German playwright Heinrich von Kleist (1777-1811). Here the bear spontaneously repels all attacks of a practiced fencer, because he is not thinking and does not want anything. He only perceives each blow in his so-being and always reacts adequately. This is *yi*: pure intention undisturbed by thought, volition, and emotion, alert and clear, never doing more than what the situation requires. The Taiji master Wu Yuxiang says in the Taiji classics, "If you direct all movements through the mind in this way, your ordinary physical strength (*li*) will be transformed into spiritual power (*jin*). Then your movements will no longer be clumsy and sluggish."

The Asian martial arts all have one central goal: they want to develop inner power (*jin*) that is different from raw force (*li*). They all have in common that the main path to this power is meditative. All body movements are refined as they are guided by the focused mind, usually in combination with specific breathing techniques. The path can be compared to the refinement of steel. Iron, the raw material, is heated again and again—infused with oxygen—then artfully folded in fixed sequences of movements. In this manner, Damascus steel is produced, whose essential power is much higher than the raw strength of unprocessed ore.

This idea of refining physical strength does not exist in Western sports. For example, boxers utilize raw strength and pure force. They must get strong and learn to be skillful in various techniques. But these techniques only teach them to hit hard, raw, and uninhibited, packing punches that can kill. Boxers never learn to refine their strength; on the contrary, their goal is to break down all inhibitions when punching. To prevent this lack of restraint from causing fatal injury, their fists are packed in padded gloves.

Unlike this, Asian external martial artists use inner power to train for a victory of mind over body. With the right resilience and focus, even someone with a weak body can slice through a brick with the edge of their hand or stop a spear pressed against their chest. The Shaolin Monastery in Henan is the best-known center for this kind of practice. The skills taught there sell well in the West, where people steeped in dualistic thinking celebrate the triumph of mind over matter and admire the show of strength and technique.

True inner power in Taiji arises without this conflict of mind and body. It is free from all ego. Being free does not mean all self is forgotten in a state of bland passivity that gives in to every attack—as is misunderstood in some Taiji styles, which turn out to be dominantly external. They only know external force and do not want to use it. True power, however, preserves its own space and does not invest in losing; rather, it bounces the opponent and negates his attack.

Inner power arises from the mind. A Taiji classic says, "Rely on the mind, not the *qi*." If the mental impulse is right and the idea of the movement you have decided on is clear and distinct, then the movement will succeed and inner power will grow. If the mental impulse is not right and is unclear or incomplete, then the movement can only be brought to an end with external force. The use of raw external force ensures a movement with reluctance, protest and resistance, which causes pain for those involved. Whoever exerts the greater force wins. A defense with inner power, on the other hand, uproots the opponent and sends him flying without any feelings of pressure or pain. It is friendly and pleasant for everyone involved—it works with happy *qi*.

All this means is that the ability of a real Taiji master is not magical or esoteric: it is just a spirit-led movement of intention in a state of a trans-sensing. True inner power is subtler than raw force and penetrates the cracks and weaknesses of gross muscular strength. In the end, the weak overcomes the strong.

Qi Flow

The Taiji classics emphasize that legs and hips form the basis of the development of inner power. This is so because they are closer to the ground than arms and torso. *Qi* rises from the legs and hips, connects to breathing in the torso, and transforms into power in the arms and hands.

Qi power needs optimal body tone. Practitioners of the external martial arts tend to produce too much internal tension. They root and guide the breath as we do in internal Taiji, but they also tighten their muscles: yang energy predominates. Adepts of some Taiji styles who have not understood true inner power tend to keep inner tension too low. They are often loose and limp, and seek success only in evasion and weak movements, being effectively powerless: yin energy outweighs all else. The optimal body tone, that is, true inner power, means being firm but not rigid, soft but not yielding.

The structure of the entire body—bones, muscles, and all its dynamics—should be self-supporting in the practice Taiji. It should be as if the body were made of individual glass cylinders: not connected to each other, they can rotate freely. Another image is that of a string of coins or pearls: each joint should be able to move freely as if it were not connected to anything else, yet each link is in fact connected to the other.

Internal Taiji works with *qi* as it flows through the entire body. In contrast to Western methods such as physical therapy, it never deals with tense body parts or injured joints directly. Rather it insists that the whole body should move in such a way that the joints open by themselves and *qi* can flow freely. The body does the work on its own—all therapy is only to support its self-healing process.

Taiji movements round out the body, that is, the sequence of movements is designed so that joints open naturally as and when it is performed correctly. The body is only stretched and tensed as necessary for optimal *qi* flow in the meridians. Extreme movements, even if anatomically and physiologically possible, are consistently avoided in Taiji, and the practice never overtaxes the body. Rather, it leads gently to an optimal realignment, with neither too much nor too little tension.

This has different effects on different practitioners. Some students have to learn to let go and relax more; others are too lax and have to build up more inner tension. But the effect is the same: after practicing everyone feels better and lighter in body and mind. In sum:

> Stillness of mind and body posture gather *qi* in the center.
> Body movements and breath allow it to circulate.
> Round and expansive movements create space for *qi* and breath; they free the joints.
> The muscles serve this purpose.

Liberated joints enable health and *qi* power.

The integrated tension of the entire body does not work with the isolated tension of individual muscles, but with a tonic (Feldenkrais) or eutonic (Glaser) tension among all parts. As the muscles remain relaxed, inner power comes from the elastic interaction of all.

This holds also true for other disciplines. In archery, for example, it is crucial to find elastic tension to the point that *qi* can flow freely through the joints and the meridians remain open. The arm muscles are not contracted, the shoulders are relaxed, and the neck in its loose rotation forms a spiral. With the right breathing, *qi* can find its way out unhindered and guide the arrow to the target. If an archer stiffens and tenses his muscles without elasticity, he cannot succeed. Thus, in Zen, archery is also a path to internal cultivation (Herrigel 2003).

Inner power works without harshness or strong effort. For example, let us assume someone holds my right wrist at eye level and twists it so that my thumb points down. Normally he would be in the stronger position while I would respond with pressure and try to wriggle my arm out, using force and contorting myself. Going loose and limp in a Taiji mode will not be efficient in this situation, because dodging only works when facing an active attack, not a static hold.

Using Taiji in this situation, I respond by using inner power. I leave the arm initially to the opponent, and instead of launching a counterattack, I shape myself. I round my arms and body so the joints are open internally, then move around the grip, like a snake winding itself around a branch. Inner power arises from the interplay of the body's energy spirals and gently rolls over the opponent's grip through the interaction of *yi*, *qi*, and *jin*. The opponent does not feel any counterpressure until it is too late. He either has to loosen his grip or be thrown off balance and uprooted.

A Taiji movement with inner power is easy for the performer: free from compulsion, it is highly effective. People's typical reaction is: "But I didn't do anything!" That is because they have no feedback since they do not feel an active counterpressure, which normally reports back on the degree of force we exert. The light, twisting movement is not felt strongly, yet it compels the opponent to let go: it stuns more than it causes pressure or pain. Because the other assumes a position of force while I softly and subtly penetrate his cracks, he unexpectedly finds himself in a weak position.

Attaining the lightness of inner power is very difficult. It requires years of practice and great mental persistence. You have to learn to stay with yourself and your movement, even when an external force is active. Only when *qi* flows smoothly and the mind is aligned can the *jin* power unfold. Unfortunately, there is no everyday experience of this gentle force we could use for comparison. Over time, a physical certainty comes and you feel what the right way of not doing is like. Then the ability to use inner power accelerates and skill increases. In the end, you apply it spontaneously and with relish in any situation, coming to play with it.

The force field established through the correct interplay of spirit, breath, and movement resembles a water fountain. From the outside, the jets of water rising up and falling down appear light and floating, but they easily tumble anyone who steps in their midst.

In a very similar way, Taiji movements consist of the constant alternation of a rising energy moving toward the sky and a falling energy sinking toward the ground. The effect is also similar: the old Taiji masters let their attackers simply bounce off at the first touch, tumbling them upon contact.

Qi and Breath

The Chinese word *qi* has two main meanings. It indicates the breath, i. e., the air we breathe in and out, and also the life energy that circulates through the meridians. The two are closely interrelated in that they that indicate core potencies of life. *Qi* as life energy only circulates in beings that breathe; only where *qi* flows does a living being breathe. In a broader sense, *qi* is also the primary substance of all living things, including the planet, the stars, and the greater universe.

Breathing connects the outside world with the inside of the body. The body absorbs new *qi* when inhaling and releases used or stale *qi* upon exhalation. The meridians have acupuncture points that allow access to internal and external energy circuits. They are openings right below the skin that allow an exchange with cosmic *qi* when needled, lasered, or massaged. The body is a microcosm and thus just as much an energy system as the macrocosm of the universe. Both exchange information and affect each other constantly. Optimal harmony between them affords peace, health, and spiritual attainment.

Internal Taiji is all about true breath, an inner form of breathing that involves the whole body, works through the cells of the skin, and is often also called pore breathing.

How does this work? Normally, people move about never minding how they breathe. Although the breath naturally reacts to certain body movements from time to time, the two are not coordinated. True breath means that we coordinate breathing and body movements in such a way that each movement brings about a particular way of breathing.

As the body sinks in spirals down toward the earth, directing *qi* as life energy down and out, the mouth releases *qi* as breath in an exhalation. When the body straightens up toward the sky, *qi* moves up and in, and the lungs fill with breath in an inhalation. Depending on the type of breathing, the yin and yang phases of the form become phases of inhaling and exhaling, of drawing and releasing life energy. This covers the entire body: as Zhuangzi says, sages breathe all the way to their heels.

All martial artists coordinate movement with breath, but not in the same way. Masters of the external martial arts utilize the breath to develop raw physical force and thus willingly huff and puff, gasp and pant. Those versed in the internal martial arts like Taiji, on the other hand, are never out of breath because they know how to use gravity. Internal Taiji allows the breathing to happen without any conscious or volitional effort. The breath follows the *qi* pulse that rises and falls in relation to the ground. When the body sinks, it lets go just like the breath; when it rises, the lungs absorb the impulse and expand. The inner cycle of the breath adapts to the outer cycle of movement: both support each other. This is how the heavenly cycle or microcosmic orbit of *qi* through the body is created, and true breath comes to flow.

In order for inner power to unfold, Taiji practitioners must avoid any movement that disturbs the true breath. The biggest factor of disruption is voluntary and intentional muscle tension, a form of brute force that impacts the torso, so that the breath can no longer vibrate freely. In Daoist terms, arms must be empty and not filled with hard force.

An empty arm, however, is not a soft or limp arm that dangles in an uncoordinated manner. Rather, it is filled with *qi*. The natural tone of the fascia, which maintains the arm's shape, is not disturbed by contraction in any form: thus, breath and life energy can flow freely and inner power grows.

Breathing Types

True inner breath expresses itself in two ways, depending on the body type. Inhalers tend to work with reverse breathing, contracting the stomachs on inhalation and thus filling their lungs to develop inner power. Exhalers use abdominal breathing, expanding into the belly, and grow inner power on exhalation.

The theory of breathing types was first formulated by the musician Erich Wilk. An avid violin student and equipped with exceptional powers of observation and sensitivity, he noticed that his teachers used two major modes with regard to the breath and expressed this in terms of two different types of breathing. Later he successfully applied his knowledge in the medical and therapeutic field.

He published his discovery in 1949, also reflecting his war experience. Serving in the Afrika Korps, he a prisoner of war for three years in a rather hot climate. He noticed that, despite his good constitution, he could not stand the extreme heat and dryness, while other prisoners coped much better. In addition to these different effects of the sun on people, he also observed the effect of the moon on his violin playing and came to the conclusion that individual breathing types are connected to the sun or the moon. Next, he discovered that the dominance of sun or moon at the time of birth could be related to the evolving type. If solar energy predominated at birth, the person would be an exhaler; if lunar energy was greater, the child grew up as an inhaler.

After the war, he continued to develop his system in cooperation with the pediatrician Charlotte Hagena, who had recovered from a serious illness applying breath work. Over a period of forty years, they tested the concept of breathing types in their practice and identified diverse health-promoting behaviors for each type, primarily involving diet and exercise. They patented their system under the name terlusollogy—a term that combines the Latin words for earth, sun, and moon: *terra, sol, luna*. Today, the system is used primarily by body therapists, Yoga teachers, midwives, speech therapists, voice coaches, singers, public speakers, actors—and Taiji masters such as myself.

People of the two breathing types differ in posture, movements, vocalization, and body habits. They are also different in terms of energetic posture, which means that their activation of the true breath is not the same. Photographs and documents of eminent Taiji masters show clearly how they function differently, but this has never been systematically explored. One example is my teacher's master Yang Shouzhong who was an exhale, unlike my teacher Chu King-Hung who is an inhaler. It took Master Chu a very long time to change his teacher's form in such a way that it was a source for his own inner power. As I train my students, I take great care to identify their breathing type, facilitating their unique quest and expression as they pay close attention to just how *qi* works within them.

Lunar inhalers naturally assume an energetic posture that looks like an inverted cone standing on its tip. They draw *qi* and breathe up from a point on the feet. The higher the *qi* rises, the wider the spirals become. It moves up along the inside of the legs and into the lower `, then fills it and continues along the spine to the top of the head. This process is supported by leaning back slightly in the area of the lower lumbar spine, near the Gate of Life. This allows the breath to fills the back and chest without raising the sternum. As it continues to rise, moreover, the chin lifts slightly and the head tilts back a bit, so that the crown of the head is points straight at heaven or the sky. The arms perform an internal rotation, that is, are in pronation, and support the ascending, widening *qi* movement with relaxed muscle tone. *Jin* power spirals upward like a hydraulic system and reaches its climax at the end of the inhalation.

Inhalers pause for a short moment before starting to exhale. If an opponent grabs their arm at the very end of this breathing pause, even a tiny, easy movement of the arm, rotating it outward in a spiral, suffices to uproot them and causes them to fall, no matter how tightly they hold on. Of course, the outward spiraling of the arms is only the end point of a movement of the entire body wheel, which begins in the feet, continues as an outer spiral along the legs, effects a shift in the center (as guided by the attention), and finally translated into the arms.

Inhalers release the breath they have collected in the yin phase and never should actively exhale, lest the pelvic muscles contract. In this mode of exhaling, the *qi* descends along the front of the body back into the lower abdomen and slides down the outside of the legs into the ground.

Unlike this, solar exhalers naturally assume an energetic posture that looks like a regular cone, that is, standing on its flat side. Most striking is their pelvic position: they keep it slightly tilted so that the tailbone protrudes. This tilt comes from the Gate of Life, while the pelvis is relaxed and hangs down with ease. Upon exhalation, in exhalers *qi* moves down and spreads out. Their arms and legs spiral inward, sides and chest tighten. The lower abdomen fills with *qi*, which rotates toward the ground, and inner power grows.

They reach the peak of power at the end of their exhalation, when they have a short pause before inhaling again. If pinned, they use *jin* power on exhaling, which uproots the opponent and causes him to fall—like a stone thrown across a pond.

Exhalers do not actively inhale, but let the breath come in effortlessly, supported by outward spirals in the legs and arms as well as movements in the area of the Gate of Life. *Qi* rises from the ground along the front of the body and sinks back down along the back into the lower elixir field. From there a new heavenly cycle can begin.

The two breathing types are opposite in how they develop inner power: solar exhalers develop it when they empty the lungs, while the lunar inhalers are strongest when they fill them. The dichotomy corresponds to the principle of yin and yang: both together make up the Taiji.

In internal Taiji, victory—affording the opponent the opportunity to defeat himself—comes about without fighting or moral rules because the fight is empty and free from intentionality. It is won in a friendly manner without anyone trying to be particularly nice. Inner power is empty and formless but it works. The Yang-style master Chen Weiming describes it:

> Many people practice Taiji today, but not it the real Taiji. . . . With true Taiji, your arm is like iron wrapped in cotton. It is very soft yet feels heavy to someone trying to lift it. . . .
>
> When you touch the opponent, your hands are soft and light, but he cannot get rid of them. Your attack is like a bullet going straight through something (*gancui*)—without the help of "sluggish power." If pushed ten feet, he feels a little movement but no power. And he feels no pain. (Chen 1928, cited in Draeger and Smith 1978)

13

The Daoist Perspective

by

Emanuel Seitz

The Perfected

> The perfect man is without self;
> The spirit man is without ability;
> The sage is without name.
> —*Zhuangzi* 1.3

Daoism is a philosophy of life in search of true humanity. Perhaps we have not really understood with modern science what it means when we say: humans are living beings. All living beings are alive, yet their existence comes in different degrees and modes of aliveness.

There is the exuberant aliveness of children when they laugh and jump and frolic, overflowing with vitality and *joie de vivre*, running around to exhaustion. There is the purposeful, strenuous, and dogged life of adults who want to save their energy and shape their being. And there is an aliveness that peeks out from the sparkling and twinkling eyes of the old. Each age has its own way of being fresh, pliable, and limber.

Opposite signs are harbingers of a declining, ebbing vitality. Sallow staring into emptiness, bloated limpness, cold rigidity, indolence, listless apathy, and ashen-gray withered skin that hangs off the bones—those are the markers of death, misfortune, and disease.

Being vitally and vibrantly alive is more important to human beings than bare physical existence. Not everything that prolongs life also maintains vitality, but that is what counts —it determines destiny and the quality of existence.

Daoists focus strongly on the task of cultivating vitality. They understand each and every kind of life as a form of *qi*, the cosmic life force and energy that manifests to different degrees and strengths. To put it figuratively, Daoists think of living entities as having an innate energy balance, sort of like a battery that can be depleted or recharged. Cables and circuits run through it to allow *qi* to flow, and there are various transformers to convert and adjust the voltage. However, this is how far the image of the battery goes: *qi* as vital energy is not limited to the electromagnetic waves of physics and communications technology. It is about the pure power of life, a vibrant force, the core energy of the universe.

The highest dimension of this living force of *qi* is spiritual in nature. It creates spooky long-distance effects. People who, after long periods of practice, have become clear in their heart and mind, confident in their speech, and well expressed in their appearance, reach a level of efficacious vitality that is beyond the visible. They exude a charisma, something immense and uncanny, a mood, an aura.

What seems astonishing or even miraculous to ordinary folk, happens easily, spontaneously, and casually in such people. They possess the effortless flexibility of children, the creative determination of adults, and the unshakable calm of the elderly. Full of inner power, they make an impression, even when it is dormant and they are ostensibly not doing very much. Daoists call this inner power *de*, often translated "virtue." It represents the living force that arises directly from Dao, the potency of the universal way.

They call people imbued with this power perfected (*zhenren*) or sages (*shengren*), either term indicating superior human beings who have the dignity of saints. Representing a level of aliveness that is the ultimate goal of all, they live in harmony with their own so-being and the nature of the world. Capable of attaining immortality, they serve as role models for all humanity and in their power continue to shine, affecting others even after they depart from this planet.

In a more religious dimension, Daoists posit the existence of gods (*shen*) and immortals (*xian*), superior people who are deified, revered, and worshiped. But wisdom, perfection, and immortality are not the result of supernatural grace. There is no gift, nothing is bestowed by an otherworldly, supernatural being. No god chooses them as saints and holy men. The core of Daoism, despite supporting a vast pantheon, is deeply atheistic and even materialistic in its spirituality. Salvation and enlightenment come after long practice and are the result of slow and patient work on oneself that transforms body and spirit. Seekers purify, refine, and cultivate themselves until they are filled with calm simplicity. Sages live with ease on this earth, always from clarity and stillness, strong and invisible like the wind. The perfected rest within themselves like the eye of a hurricane.

Nourishing Life

> Yours truly prefers to utilize Dao.
> It is more than skill.
> —Zhuangzi 3.2

Daoism is a way of life that is good for nothing and good for everything. In Chinese, its central concern for physical health and long life is called nourishing life (*yangsheng*). Just like a mother breastfeeding her child or a gardener watering flowers, people should take care of themselves. Reading the term literally, it is quite absurd, as it refers to something that is actually impossible. Life cannot be fed; it has nothing to feed on. Rather, the word "nourish" indicates the idea of benevolent care. Mother and gardener do not want anything from their charges: they do not expect wages or rewards but only care about creating the best possible conditions so the life entrusted to them can unfold fully. They remove anything harmful and provide the right nourishment, thus encouraging vigorous growth as much as possible.

In the same way, people should take good care of their bodies and lives, they should be gentle, kind, and nurturing toward themselves. To ensure their continued existence, they must direct their attention to the self-evident forces that enliven them and promote their vitality. To this end, Daoists developed a plethora of ideas and practices—proper breathing, healthful diet, healing exercises, environmental regulation (Fengshui), mental discipline, emotional restraint, and moderation in all activities. For millennia, they have devoted themselves to the question how human beings can best preserve and enhance their lives. Taiji, Qigong, and various forms of meditation all form part of this program to promote vitality. They enhance inner power and maintain health: their ultimate goal is none other than life itself.

Daoists in their pursuit of nourishing life, unlike Westerners, never seek a reason for well-being in an external purpose of existence. They prolong life and enhance health by avoiding harmful things and teaching people the art of flowing through life with ease. They insist on strengthening the steadfastness of character, yet always leave it up to the individual to set their own goals. They serve life and do not transform it into the servant of a higher, transcendent purpose.

It may be wise to have a purpose for one's existence, a scheme that gives order and direction to life, protecting it from aimless wandering and running around. Having a purpose provides meaning to existence, a reason for action to the mind, and the hope for improvement to one's thinking. But really good times have the disadvantage of never actually being there in the present moment.

People keep on envisioning and betting on a future that is not yet there. At its worst, hope is the reason why they sacrifice their present life—accepting miserable conditions as the price they have to pay for a better future. As wonderful as their goals may be, there is the great danger that they waste a good part of their lives and their selves. They run after the farthest, most exalted goals and at the same time make themselves dependent on compulsive ideas, never ceasing to be fooled by randomness.

All external goals have the same weakness: people have no safe control over their realization. This realization depends on outside circumstances, personal destiny, and the goodwill of others. There is always something artificial and contrived about such goals, something ultimately shallow and untrue. They take away freedom, since people's entire lives are dedicated to them.

Also, they create artificial structures: when everything only follows one purpose and serves one meaning, nothing happens by itself, spontaneously, or naturally. It does not matter whether the goal is realistic or fantastic. People ruin their lives on earth for an imaginary salvation in heaven; they live only for duty and honor to create a utopian world. A shift in consciousness toward a more Daoist way of being, therefore, means that they must no longer use life as a means for external purposes and idealistic plans.

A good antidote to such purposeful thinking and a life dedicated to external goals is the Daoist doctrine of the usefulness of the useless. The *Zhuangzi* tells the story of a gnarled, old tree with branches so wide that entire herds of cattle could graze in their shade. The tree gained its humongous growth and extensive longevity only because it was useless as timber: its stem and branches were twisted and crooked. Because it was useless, it could go on living. Then, however, once it had reached the fullness of life, its uselessness became useful in its own way: the huge branches spread shade and gave respite to beast and man (4.5-6).

In the same manner, Daoists support all sorts of apparently useless longevity practices as useful concerns for life. The same also applies to the search for immortality: life by necessity moves toward death, which means that any worry about living forever is by necessity vain and pointless. However, striving for this essentially useless goal has a useful benefit: it leads people to improve their well-being and ensures that they live with greater aliveness, even if they never actually make it to immortality. Nourishing life does not add meaning to life, and yet it is not meaningless.

This concern for one's own existence creates the conditions for being able to live in harmony with Dao. To Daoists, the world is vibrantly alive, continuously becoming and passing away. Each and every form of existence is constantly swallowed up by nothingness if destiny so wills, without any higher meaning above and behind the ongoing processes of birth and death, rise and decline. The primary purpose of life is to live, to continue one's existence, and enhance well-being. Finitude is part of its nature and makes up its essence, but its higher truth manifests in lived activity. Every life works in the world.

If people really want to nourish life and not just sustain it, that is, cultivate it and let it grow, they must realize their full potential and acquire relevant skills to the point where they can increase their effectiveness. Daoists live in a culture of daily practice, realizing their true self though selfless ability. Sages are always free from self since they align all their activities with Dao and do not follow their personal likes and dislikes. Being deeply rooted in Dao, they have superior abilities beyond common competence and dexterity. They have transformed their self to a great level of mastery that amazes everyone. Masters who know how to use Dao work in all venues of life: cooks, carpenters, warriors, poets, and more— it makes no difference. Everything to them becomes a way of nurturing life.

Dao and World

> The way that moves is not the eternal way.
> The name that names is not the eternal name.
> —Daodejing 1

Daoism is the philosophy of Dao. The term *dao* means "way" and, used as a verb, indicates walking when things are going well and running when they are going smoothly. It signifies both, a path and movement along it, indicating the process of walking and doing along a given trajectory plus the artistry or accomplishment that come at the end of a long journey.

Dao leads to a development that increases power and competence, authority and dominion. A military general, for example, works with Dao as he follows his training manual that gives instructions on how to become a warrior and strategist. Being a warrior does not mean—as Westerners might think—being accomplished and complete, polished and competent after completing a certain curriculum. A perfect warrior who works with Dao is fully present in each and every activity; he constantly pursues what makes him a good soldier. Perfection is new every day: there is no superiority without constant rehearsing and staying in motion. One does the best one can: things will go well if and when they are supposed to do so.

Daoists have adopted the term *dao*, traditionally used to describe a way of training and expertise, and raised it to denote the core power of the world. To them, all in the universe is Dao—a walk, a way, a positive movement of life. This movement or ongoing process is the only constant on earth; it constitutes its essence. Change and transformation are at the core and the pinnacle of the world, its outstanding and distinguishing characteristics. Everything constantly moves forward, arises and declines, ultimately finite and transitory.

Dao has five features or principles that characterize its structure. The first is that the world originates in nonbeing (*wu*) and returns there. Dao is like an empty circle or wheel that is constantly turning and is without beginning or end. Its motion is uncreated, not willed by any god. It simply is: *creatio continua*. Constantly bringing forth and destroying, it gives life to all beings in the world from nonbeing and causes them to disappear again into nonbeing. Such origin means both, that the world has a beginning and that this beginning is not absolute.

All beginnings in this world arise of themselves from the perpetual free play of arising and passing away. Unifying and concentrating dynamics alternate with those dissolving and scattering. All things, human and other living beings, come from the indefinite and formless, and eventually fall back into it. Formless and faceless chaos (*hundun*) is the origin of all that is. Everything is mixed up in it, like the filling of a dumpling floating in soup. Death is nothing but a return to indeterminacy. The orderly dissolves, rots, decays, and turns back into a formless mass, into the nonbeing it was before its birth.

Even the end of the world in the Daoist universe is nonbeing. There are goals, directions, inclinations, and tendencies, but there is no ultimate goal. What happens in the world is not entirely chaotic and disorderly, but on the whole the world is on a course toward nonbeing. It moves forward, it transforms, but there ultimately no whence and whither.

The second major principle of Dao is the quality of change and transformation which works with the "alternation of opposites." The world unfolds due to the activity of two forces in constant conflict and mutual complementation—yin and yang. The terms refer to modes of energetic action, describing what happens to an entity in the course of time, how and when it changes. Yin indicates the tendency toward compression and absorption: it signals energy moving inward. Yang marks the trend toward release and dissolution: it indicates energy moving outward. All phenomena of the world match this scheme, understood as part of an energy cycle or exchange.

By and large, these two forces work closely with each other, preventing the world from descending into chaos. However, there are frequent imbalances that lead to deficiency or excess on one side or the other. They result in blockages, diseases, and natural disasters—in other words, all those phenomena that cause the otherwise smooth running of the world to falter

Third, Dao represents the inherent unity of the world, linked an essential feature that remains indeterminable and incomprehensible. As the scriptures say, it is formless (*wuxing*) and nameless (*wuming*), called *dao* only because there is no precise term. This appellation "way" or "path" is ultimately only a proxy for something quite beyond human comprehension.

Being formless and nameless, Dao commands without laws and rules. If becoming had rules, one could define it, understand it, make sense of it, and use it for one's own ends. It is, of course, possible to elicit certain laws and regular patterns from nature, to learn how the natural processes function and which factors work together. With such insight, the natural patterns can be put to use and serve human purposes. Modern science is one result of this: people become the ruler of nature by examining and obeying its laws. Francis Bacon (1561-1626), the inventor of the empirical natural sciences in the West, formulated this principle in his *Novum Organon* of 1620: "Nature is not conquered except by obedience" (*Natura non nisi parendo vincitur*).

However, the Daoist relation to nature is not geared toward ruling it. There are plenty of laws and rules, regular patterns and structural organizations, but they should be followed and enjoyed rather than obeyed and subdued. Formless and nameless at its core, Dao has a certain degree of unpredictability, a deep uncertainty in becoming. Its actions elude plans and defy human imagination, yet the patterns of yin and yang are discernible and can serve as guidelines to behaviors that lead to health, harmony, and prosperity.

The fourth principle of Dao is that it is self-sustaining and represents the free and unlimited play of various forces, neither a mechanism nor an organism. There is no firm, set, or rigid system in this world. It is not a closed, predetermined structure with different functions, organs, or machine parts. As described in the texts, it is more like a strategy game where the goal is the balance of power. The whole is preserved and remains intact as long as no part becomes too strong or too weak, if energy circulates and the cycle is not disrupted.

For example, in Chinese medicine, the organs are not doing the work, but the particular form of *qi* that emanates from them. They connect to other forms of *qi* that arise on the outside, such as breath and food, weather and seasons, social institutions and human communities. All these forms morph according to their weight and power in each overall situation. Disease is caused by the deficiency or excess of certain forms of *qi* that weaken the body's defensive energy (*weiqi*). Invading microbes are not the ultimate cause: rather, a weakness in the immune system allows bacteria or viruses to take over the body.

The dominant Daoist focus on worldly phenomena as continuously changing situations leads to a great concern for knowledge about how something works and how different effects interact. It is not conducive to a search for one single element, one main active ingredient, or one key factor that is the cause of everything. There may be a core pivot in the system that turns everything on, but it is not the subject of inquiry. Traditional Chinese thinkers know that things work, but they are not very interested to find out a single reason why. Rather, they see patterns of functioning in the dynamic interplay of forces, energies, physical entities, and intentions. Their explanations do not look for roots but express and structure discernible dynamic effects and the interplay of forces.

When Daoists nourish life, they accordingly aim to maintain the dynamic balance of the life forces. Rather than fighting a disease that is already manifest, they look to health maintenance and prevention. They know how to create balance between the different forces, so that people can remain strong and integrated in themselves. Their main focus is to take care of Dao, to ensure that things run smoothly in the ongoing process of change and transformation. If one resists the changing world, one gets weak, is worn down, and eventually destroyed. As and when one adapts to change, one can retain and even grow one's power through the dynamics of life and gains the ability to sustain it without harm over long periods. In harmony with Dao, one consumes little and can become immortal.

Fifth and finally, Dao is soft and weak, bland and insipid, silent and obscure. As the *Daodejing* says, the highest effectiveness is not in the hard, but in the soft. Vigorous and loud heroes fall when they meet resistance; calm and quiet anti-heroes meet no resistance and thus save their lives and have more far-reaching effects.

The effectiveness of Dao can be compared to water: it is supple and does not remain in one position, it can transform and make detours, it nestles and yet exerts constant pressure, hollowing every stone that stands in its way through many tiny and subtle effects. At the same time, it benefits everyone and does not favor anyone—just like the sound of a blade of grass growing has a subtle effect.

Classical Thinkers

> But do we not only praise the wise,
> whose name is emblazoned on the book!
> For one must first snatch his wisdom from the wise.
> Therefore, the customs officer should also be thanked:
> He asked for it.
> —Bertold Brecht (1898-1958), German playwright

There are three major thinkers of classical Daoist thought: Laozi, Zhuangzi, and Liezi, whose works are key sources of both religious and philosophical Daoism. Laozi's *Daodejing*, the "Book of Dao and Its Potency," is the earliest among them. It was compiled on the basis of the teachings of a figure known by the honorary name Laozi, which literally means Old Master. He was also called Lao Dan, Old Long Ears, which refers to the ancient Chinese idea that long ears were a sign of wisdom.

Historical records describe him as a man named Li Er who lived in the 6th century BCE and served the Zhou royal court as an archivist. The story goes that he deplored the decline of the dynasty and decided to emigrate, riding west on a water buffalo. On a border pass, later located to the Zhongnan mountains southwest of modern Xi'an and today marked by the Louguantai Monastery, the border guard Yin Xi stopped him and demanded that he dictate his wisdom. Laozi transmitted the work in 5000 characters and moved on—according to other, later sources to "convert the barbarians" and create Buddhism.

The standard edition of the text today goes back to the commentary by Wang Bi (226-249 CE). Even before then, the text was divided into eighty-one chapters of aphoristic verses and two parts: the first part (chs. 1-37) deals with Dao and the second (chs. 38-81) with potency. An earlier version was discovered in 1973 in a tomb at Mawangdui near Changsha, Hunan. Dated to 168 BCE, it consisted of several silk manuscripts, in which the order of the two parts is reversed, placing life application before cosmic speculation. Even before then, the bamboo slips unearthed at Guodian, also in Hunan, date back to the 4th century BCE and contain about one third of the later text.

The *Daodejing* is a classic book of wisdom. The frequently rhyming sentences and aphorisms are easy to remember and, like proverbs, have become part of the cultural Chinese heritage. The work originally served as advice to rulers who wanted to learn methods of good governance, while at the same time imparting mystical insights into the nature of the world. Its fundamental outlook is a sort of essential liberalism. The ruler should not interfere with the tasks of his ministers and subjects, so that all around him can develop freely and fulfill their natural potential, working and acting in accordance with their own nature.

The central teaching is "acting without action" (*wuwei*), a way of being in the world that does not interfere with the natural course of things and thus achieves its purpose. It is a way of acting that does not impose one's will on other beings or situations. Do what is needed without fanfare: it will feel as if you do nothing. This is how perfected and sages function in the world—they work no differently than Dao itself.

The *Zhuangzi* is a text in thirty-three prose chapters that was named after its main contributing thinker. Zhuang Zhou lived in the 3rd century BCE and worked as overseer in a lacquer garden. His disciples recorded his works as well as those of several other early Daoist figures in this collection, which survives also in a 3rd-century CE edition, revised by the thinker Guo Xiang (d. 312). Later venerated as a sacred text, it was given the honorary title *Nanhua zhenjing* (Perfect Book of Southern Efflorescence).

The *Zhuangzi* expresses many concepts found in the *Daodejing* in parables and stories. What Laozi only hints at, Zhuangzi transforms into grand allegories and symbolic anecdotes. The usefulness of the useless, the effectiveness of the perfected, the relationship to established teachers such as Confucius, and the return to the original simplicity of an uncarved block all have become immortal images of world literature.

The third major early text is the *Liezi*, similarly named after its author, Lie Yukou, and later called by the honorary title *Chongxu zhenjing* (Perfect Book of Simplicity and Vacuity). Mentioned in the *Zhuangzi* as an immortal who rides on the wind and, as a perfected, is no longer bound to the transience of the body, Liezi lived in the 4th century BCE, but his work was lost and only reconstituted in the 4th century CE by the commentator Zhang Zhan. This work is the most cosmological among the three: it has much in common with the *Zhuangzi*, replicating and expanding numerous stories.

In addition to these three, there are large numbers of later works, collected in the Daoist Canon, which survives today in its 1445 printing plus various later supplements. They include philosophical treatises, revealed and devotional texts, ritual manuals, community rules, instructions on nourishing life, and detailed outlines of meditation methods, as well as documents on the most prevalent cultivation system since the Song dynasty, internal alchemy.

Good examples of this latter tradition appear in the *Xingming guizhi* (Pointers to Inner Nature and Destiny; Darga 1999) and the *Taiyi jinhua zongzhi* (The Secret of the Golden Flower; Wilhelm 1962). Just like the ancient thinkers who were also steeped in cultivation practices, those dedicated to the religion strive to transform themselves through a variety of techniques that ultimately lead to clarity and stillness, concentration and superiority, health and inner power. This key concern with self-transformation, especially based on the body, is where the greatest differences to Western religions appear: Easterners practice first and believe second; Westerners believe first and practice second.

Emptiness

> Nonbeing is the origin of heaven and earth.
> Being is the mother of the world.
> —*Daode jing* 1

Daoists see the return to the origins as the beginning of perfection in life. Ordinary people who worry and get sick do so because they put their efforts in the wrong direction, wasting their energy on misguided goals. They chase after wealth and position, wanting nothing more than to be an important part of a complex, hierarchical, and differentiated society. Due to these goals, they get further and further away from their true being. Caring for or nourishing life, then, begins with a turn-about of the spirit, with going back to the source of inner power, to the plain and simple.

For Daoists, origin is nonbeing—the empty center. It marks the condition, where Dao can move most freely and openly. The *Daodejing* says:

> Thirty spokes are united around the hub to make a wheel.
> But it is on its nonbeing that the utility of the carriage depends.
> Water and clay are molded to form a vessel.
> But it is on its nonbeing that the utility of the vessel depends....
> Therefore, turn being into advantage and turn nonbeing into utility.
> (ch. 11)

Emptiness affords usefulness in all sorts of things. The wheel cannot turn and carry a chariot without the open space in its hub; the vessel can only serve when it is shaped so it is empty in the middle. In the same way human beings enter a state of emptiness within when they recover the origin.

Nonbeing is the source of all subtle, effortless effects. An empty, open center rests in itself: it forms the core and the foundation of great movements and transformations. Here nothing can be seen: it remains invisible. If lost, the vessel shatters and the water spills; the chariot breaks and its cargo scatters. Without an empty center, energies lose their guidance, scatter, and do harm.

To pursue this empty center, one does not have to do more; on the contrary, one should do and be less. Distractions and involvement with outside affairs keep people from resting in this empty nonbeing which alone allows them to become their true selves.

Sages and perfected accordingly practice fasting of the heart-mind (*xinzhai*). For Daoists, the heart is the seat of all thinking and feeling, the source of all desires, cravings, and aversions. People think much too much, and intellectual beliefs and ideas often become constantly troubling motives for action. This holds also true for the general will to know and the longing for emotional connection. A random stimulus is often enough to make people devote themselves to something that seems interesting for hours, yet in the end they realize they were just passing time to avoid getting bored. Time passes of itself—keeping it is the real art.

During mind-fasting, adepts allow this boredom to happen; they direct their attention inward to observe their feelings, release their thoughts, and control their volition. With an empty heart-mind, they come to see the world as it is and not as it should be. But they have to cleanse it of all projections that cloud spirit as consciousness. With a purified heart-mind, they see the world as if through a mirror, unadulterated and without intention.

By fasting the heart-mind, sages acquire a spontaneity based on the original nature of their character. They no longer worry about how they should be, but just are who they are. They make no demands on the world or others that they should follow their wishes or desires, even though they may not be how the sages would like them to be. Sages are calm and free from all attachments to external things, to anything beyond their control. They do not lecture or convert others, interfere with natural or social processes, but quietly and simply go about their way. As they stand on their own in complete freedom from wanting and acting, they form a role model for the world, attracting people to imitate them. They acquire a charisma, an aura that resonates with Dao: potency or virtue.

There is not one type of sage, perfected, or immortal. Rather they come in all different shapes and forms, often all-too-human in their expression of their uniqueness in Dao. They may work as artisans, hunters, shop keepers, or government officials; they may be of high status or low, managers or bums, crazy or crippled, martial artists or actors. They have none of the pathos of those noble and sublime moralists who pride themselves on their virtues, engage in social affairs, and try to mold others. They do not seek power or get caught up in the business of success. Rather, as Zhuangzi says of himself, they want to live like a turtle dragging its tail in the mud (17.11). They are very real—sure of themselves as individuals yet in many ways no different from ordinary folk.

Nonaction

> Those who practice learning become more every day.
> Those who practice Dao become less every day.
> —*Daodejing* 48

Daoists teach a way of not acting that is not idle. The *Daodejing* says, "Dao rests always in nonaction, yet nothing remains undone" (ch. 64). This feature is at the essence of Dao; it characterizes the effect sages and perfected have in the world as they adapt themselves to the course of Dao.

The most powerful transformations in the world are not caused by actions. They come with no intention, aim, or purpose—they may not even come with a volition or plan. Transformations are not intentionally designed and controlled—there is not ultimate mover like God behind them, nor is there a cause that makes them happen. Yet they arise and occur. They are part of fate, destiny, necessity: imperative as they keep happening.

In Dao, everything falls into place when everyone does their own thing. In this integrated, symphonic play of forces, there are two ways in which one side can become more powerful and stronger than the other. One is the way of hardness and strength: someone hard and strong conquers another, also hard and strong, with violence. That is, they engage in the clash of two forces of the same kind, where the side that puts more mass into the collision emerges victorious.

According to the *Daodejing*, this kind of victory is rare in nature. Here the second way comes into play: the soft defeats the hard and outwits it. As soon as something is hard, it always has holes and cracks that an opponent can penetrate. The holes, like the hub of a wheel, are empty places in the thing. Their presence allows a soft force to take advantage. The soft penetrates the structure of the hard and bursts it open from within. Water is a prime example: it collects in crevices on mountains, freezes, and breaks even the hardest rock.

The victory of the soft over the hard does not succeed through major force, but utilizes the emptiness and nonbeing of the opponent. Water fills the emptiness of the rock and thus gains smooth control over its hardness. Water never attacks the rock directly, nor does it avoid it. Water persists, hugging with pressure and sticking to the rock until its strength gives way. When water freezes, it blocks all internal movements of the rock crystal and enlarges its natural cracks and crevices.

The soft is not passive, but constantly and persistently pursues a way to infiltrate the hard. It adapts to circumstances and flows along with ease;

it shapes the world and is shaped by it. The power of water manifests in all different circumstances and emerges as a force of transformation. It goes along with each situation and utilizes already existing weak points with little force. It does not want or do anything. A tiny disturbance, like the butterfly effect, produces great changes that seem to come about by themselves. In this sense, soft suppleness rests in nonaction, yet leaves nothing undone.

Daoists ideally deal with the world in this manner. When everything falls into place, things happen naturally or spontaneously (ziran), without the use of external power or harsh violence. The effect is softness and lightness, which arise when people know how to use the cracks and open spaces that make up the nonbeing of a being. From them the supreme utility of Dao grows: it works with inner power rather than outward skill. The *jin* power of Taiji accordingly eschews the use of muscular force and takes advantage of the cracks and weaknesses in the opponent's natural body structure to uproot him.

The *Zhuangzi* story of Cook Ding is a powerful illustration of this strategy. He surprises the local lord he works for because he can cut up a sacrificial ox as if it were nothing. As he then explains, his path to this mastery emerged along several stages. First, he saw only the individual animal and worked on each part and section separately. Next, he perceived the ox as a whole and recognized its inherent structures. Third and highest, he went beyond this, forgetting the specifics and letting himself be guided by the inherent nature of the beast.

Now his vital energy moves along with the Dao patterns of the creature while he forgets himself—neither resting with himself nor with the animal. His mind becomes pure spirit and functions like a mirror. He moves his knife along the natural lines of the carcass, works with the cavities between muscles and tendons, bones and flesh. His knife penetrates deep into these naturally weak points, remaining sharp and saving the strength of the cook. Cook Ding has enormous skill, finely honed over nineteen years of practice, but he goes beyond that—he flows in spirit and works with Dao. As he adapts to the natural course of things, he remains in nonaction, yet nothing remains undone (3.2).

The highest level of Daoist nonaction means that one no longer has to do anything in order to generate an effect. Another *Zhuangzi* parable tells of a man named Yi Xingzi who raises fighting cocks. It is not enough for him that they are full of strength and burst with courage. He continues to train them until they control all emotions, become unfazed by their surroundings, and look so menacing that all contenders run off. Only when their mind stops wandering is their inner power complete. Such fighting cocks show no outward weakness and have no cracks or crevices that could be penetrated. For such roosters—or people—nonaction is their true inner nature (*xing*) and destiny (*ming*) (19.9).

Yet Daoist nonaction does not mean being lazy. Rather, it is —as Martin Buber put it—the "activity of the human being who has become whole" (1983, 77). With the assimilation to Dao and the return to nature, human beings develop into an effective wholeness, which causes all their activities to happen in unity with themselves and the world. There is no more self-will in any part, only concentrated inner power and highest effectiveness.

Taiji

> He who knows does not speak;
> He who speaks does not know.
> —*Daodejing* 56

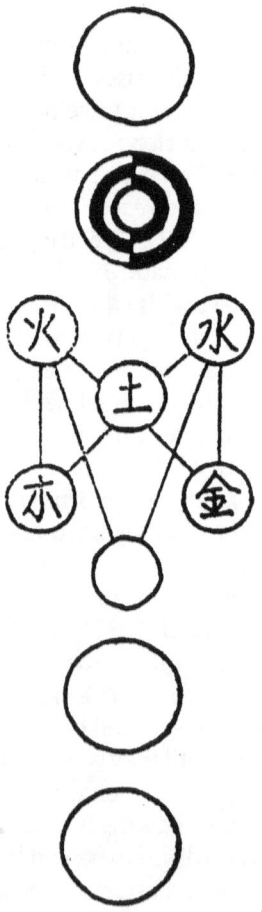

Taiji, the Great Ultimate, defined as the combined integration of yin and yang, emerges from Wuji, the Non-Ultimate. The terms combine the words for "big" or "great" (*tai*) as well as that for "nonbeing" (*wu*) with "roofbeam" or "ultimate" (*ji*) and mark the supreme underlying principles of all existence: being (*you*) arising from nonbeing (*wu*). Wuji is at the root, as the *Yijing* says, "Wuji and then Taiji" (*wuji er taiji*). The particle *er* that links the two connotes both: that nothing precedes being, and that nonbeing is still present throughout. The Great Ultimate cannot exist without the Non-Ultimate—all being always rests in nonbeing.

Various diagrams have illustrated this principle over the years. The famous *Taijitu* (Diagram of the Great Ultimate) goes back to the Confucian thinker Zhou Dunyi (1017-1073). It shows an empty circle at the top, symbolizing the Non-Ultimate, then a second circle with yin and yang rotating in black-and-white spirals around an empty core. This shows how being in all cases has nonbeing at its center and expresses itself in complementary forces. From there, the five phases emerge, that is, the world unfolds. Personal cultivation, in turn, leads back to the empty circle

Later, in the 17th century, the diagram or symbol appeared that is commonly used today: the double fish graphic of the Chinese monad, which shows a harmony of the two opposites of yin and yang (see Fig. 1 above; Bödicker 2015; Louis 2003).

The *Taijitu* combines the major principles of Chinese cosmology that serve to explain world phenomena. There is a certain tendency in this philosophy to express the abstract through images. People distrust arguments about words and prefer to show what they mean. Showing gives a view and teaches without words. Teaching without words is also the ideal of the Daoist sages.

However, just staring at an image in silence does not help—a teacher is needed to explain the principles. The hallmark of Taiji thinking, then, is that all phenomena only exist in duality, yin versus yang. Oneness or unity only occurs as a combination of converging and diverging forces, movements, or forms of *qi*. It is a constant balancing act that forever strives for harmony.

Any movement in the world runs smoothly and without disturbance as long as the opposing forces alternate flexibly and work at about the same strength. Any deviation leads to excess, deficiency, stagnation, or blockage—various ways the *qi* flow moves out of sync—and over time results in misfortune and disease. Yin and yang are complementary opposites, manifest in light and shadow, inhalation and exhalation, movement and stillness, giving and receiving, and so on. They can never be both in the same place, stand in relation to the same thing, or happen at the same time—and if there were only one and not also the other, the world would fall apart.

Daoist methods of nourishing life serve to bring order into this conflict that pervades all existence. They show how a regular exchange between the two forms of *qi* can ensure smooth flow and good circulation. The practice of Taiji sets this clear alternation between yin and yang into motion and supports an orderly flow of *qi* on the basis of a regular rhythm of giving and receiving. Without practicing this rhythm, there is only wild *qi* that is easily wasted.

The highest form of being is the alternation of opposites—not their coincidence. This vision holds true for Daoists as much as for Nicholas of Cusa and other Western mystics. The coincidence of opposites goes beyond that, into nonbeing: it is not only seen as the highest form of wisdom but also as a way of attaining the ultimate stage of return to the origin. This is the Non-Ultimate (Wuji) and not the Great Ultimate (Taiji), the gateway to the highest form of pure so-being.

This small theoretical detail is very important when dealing with yin and yang. Western thinkers tend to think of Daoists as post-modern constructivists—especially when it comes to false esotericism—who claim that there are no clear differences in the world, that all differences are blurred and ultimately dissolve in a diverse and undifferentiated flow of phenomena. This is not what Taiji is about at all—on the contrary: you first have to cultivate clear opposites before you can use them from a position of nonbeing. Sponginess is a serious misunderstanding of Far Eastern wisdom.

Nothing is gray in this teaching; everything is either white or black. The transition is a leap and not a growth or development. Even the refinement of transitions does not allow gray to emerge, but a renewed duality of yin and yang, namely yin within yang (spring) and yang within yang (summer) in the yang phase, plus yin within yin (winter) and yang within yin (autumn) in the yin phase.

The attributions are always precise once the principle is understood: Yang always gives and radiates *qi*: white, sun, heaven, and movement from inside to outside. Yin always receives and absorbs *qi*: black, moon, earth, and the movement from outside to inside. One has only to get used to thinking in terms of energies rather than substances, then the differences become clear and distinct. For advanced learners, moreover, the following holds true: nothing is not even gray in Daoism—it is colorless. Gray just does not exist. The center is empty.

Humanity

> The king follows earth,
> Earth follows heaven,
> Heaven follows Dao.
> Dao follows only itself.
> —*Daodejing* 25

Life is a daily task and a constant exercise in futility. "Life lasts because nobody could handle it," the German poet Rainer Maria Rilke says in *The Inheritance of Count C. W.* The same applies to Daoist nourishing life: caring for and nurturing inner power and vitality impart no great achievements or skills and afford only a limited mastery over destiny. The ideal of the master of life, a wise and perfect person, promises a completely different ability at the end of constant effort that cannot be measured in achievements. The ability to be oneself and be whole is the highest level of self-realization in the world. It means living in harmony with Dao.

Human beings come from the union of heaven and earth, they are of both heavenly and earthly origin. Their power manifests in the so-called three treasures: life energy (*qi*), primordial essence (*jing*), and spirit (*shen*). All three are forms of *qi* at different levels of aggregation. As taught in internal alchemy, primordial essence contains genetic material which condenses into the physical constitution, liquefies into bodily life energy, and evaporates into spirit and consciousness as which it can leave the body. Through the techniques of nourishing life, adepts learn to transform it into *qi*, then the move on to transform *qi* into spirit, as which they then can enter emptiness and nonbeing. Reaching this, they return to the origin, find their true nature, and reverse the process of world formation.

The great result of this internalized reversal of creation is the realization of skillful living. Sages, perfected, and immortals become a source in the world that creates and creates ever more. They no longer waste their time, but use their facilities and potentials to the fullest. They concentrate their energy in whatever they do, and internally direct it to transform into spirit. At the same time, their spirit is supple and combines the hard and soft in one integrated whole. They no longer do anything that goes against the nature of beings, even those oppose them, and thereby remain undamaged in their own being.

As pure spirit people (*shenren*), they are simple and self-sufficient. As the *Zhuangzi* notes, they have skin as white as snow and the grace of young girls; they breathe the wind and drink the dew, ride on clouds and are light as feathers (1.5). I do not know if full realization to this degree is possible, but the spirit of these images surely remains immortal.

References

Anders, Frieder. 1979. *Das chinesische Schattenboxen: Tai Chi* . Frankfurt: Scherz Verlag.

_____. 2003. *Das Innere Tai Chi Chuan*. Berlin: Theseus.

_____. 2015 [1985]. *Taichi: Chinas lebendige Weisheit*. Düren: Shaker.

_____Frieder. 2020. *Das Qi verwurzeln: Qigong und Atemtypen*. Heidelberg: Kristkeitz Verlag.

Bauer, Wolfgang. 1971. *China und die Hoffnung auf Glück*. Munich: Hanser.

Bödicker, Martin. 2015. *Erläuterung des Taiji-Diagramms*. Willich: CreateSpace.

Buber, Martin. 1983. *Ich und Du*. Stuttgart: Reclam.

Chua, Amy. 2011. *Battle Hymn of the Tiger Mother*. New York: Penguin.

Cleary, Thomas. 1988. *The Art of War: Sun Tzu*. Boston: Shambhala.

Darga, Martina. 1999. *Das alchemistische Buch von innerem Wesen und Lebensenergie: Xingming guizhi*. Munich: Diederichs.

Draeger, Donn F., and Robert W. Smith. 1978. *Asian Fighting Arts*. New York: Kodansha.

Dürckheim, Karlfried. 1975. *Wunderbare Katze und andere Zen Texte*. Bern: O. W. Barth.

Elias, Norbert. 1939. *Über den Prozess der Zivilisation*. Basel: Haus zum Falken.

_____. 1982. *The Civilizing Process*. Oxford: Basil Blackwell.

Eno, Robert. 2016. *Mencius: An Online Teaching Translation*. http://hdl.handle.net/2022/23421.

Feldenkrais, Moshe. 1987. *Die Entdeckung des Selbstverständlichen*. Frankfurt: Suhrkamp.

Gerhards, Marco. 2016. *Die Atemformen beim Menschen*. Saarbrücken: Neue Erde.

Grossmann-Schnyder, Moia, and Volkmar Glaser. 1998. *Psychotonik*. Stuttgart: Haug Verlag.

Gruen, Arno. 1990. *Verrat am Selbst*. Munich: dtb

Hagena, Charlotte, and Christian Hagena. 1997. *Konstitution und Bipolarität: Erfahrungen mit einer neuen Typenlehre*. Heidelberg: Haug Verlag.

Hasegawa, Yoshiya. 2019. *Daumen-Yoga für das Gehirn*. Munich: Goldmann Verlag.

Hauskeller, Michael. 2004. *Ich denke, aber bin ich?* Munich: C. H. Beck.

Jullien, François. 1999. *Über die Wirksamkeit*. Berlin: Merve Verlag.

———. 2004. *A Treatise on Efficacy: Between Western and Chinese Thinking*. Honolulu: University of Hawaii Press.

Lahm, Philipp. 2002. *Gesund kann jeder*. Munich: Südwest Verlag.

Libet, Benjamin. 1985. "Unconscious Cerebral Initiative and the Role of Conscious Will in Voluntary Action." *Behavioral and Brain Sciences* 8:529-66.

Louis, Francois. 2003. "The Genesis of an Icon: The Taiji Diagram's Early History." *Harvard Journal of Asiatic Studies* 63:145-96.

Lu, Kuan-yü. 1991 [1964]. *The Secrets of Chinese Meditation: Self-Cultivation by Mind Control as Taught in the Ch'an, Mahayana, and Taoist Schools in China*. York Beach: Samuel Weiser.

Moegling, Klaus. 2009. *Tai Chi im Test der Wissenschaft*. Cologne: Prolog-Verlag.

Möller, Hans-Georg. 2001. *In der Mitte des Kreises*. Frankfurt: Verlag der Weltreligionen.

Moore, Robert, and Douglas Gillette. 1990. *King, Warrior, Magician, Lover: Rediscovering the Archetypes of the Mature Masculine*. San Francisco: HarperSanFrancisco.

———. 2014. *König, Krieger, Magier, Liebhaber: Die Stärken des Mannes*. Hamburg: Aurinia Verlag.

Mühlhausen, Corinna, and Peter Wippermann. 2013. *Healthstyle 2 – Ein Trend wird erwachsen: Das Zeitalter der Selbstoptimierer*. Hamburg: New Business Verlag.

Postman, Neil. 1988. *We Amuse Ourselves to Death*. Frankfurt: S. Fischer.

Schleichert. Hubert. 1990., *Klassische chinesische Philosophie*. Frankfurt: Klostermann.

Smullyan, Raymond M. 2000. *Das Tao ist Stille*. Frankfurt: S. Fischer.

Unschuld, Paul U. 2009. *What Is Medicine? Western and Eastern Approaches to Healing*. Translated by Karen Reimers. Berkeley: University of California Press.

———. 2003. *Was ist Medizin? Westliche und Ostliche Wege der Heilkunst*. Munich: C. H. Beck.

Wile, Douglas. 1996. *Lost Tai-Chi Classics from the Late Ch'ing Dynasty*. Albany: State University of New York Press.

Yang, Chengfu. 2005. *The Essence and Applications of Taijiquan*. Translated by Louis Swaim, Berkeley: North Atlantic Books.

The Authors

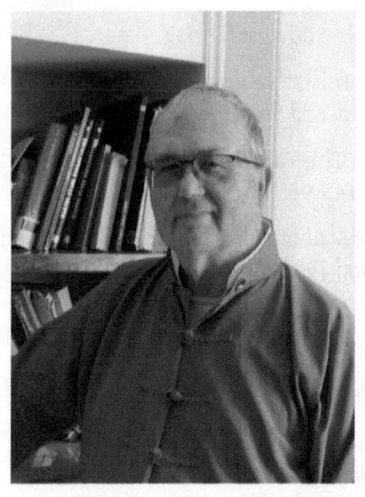

Frieder Anders (b. 1944), grandmaster of Taiji, is one of the most famous teachers in Europe. A practitioner since 1973, he worked with the key masters both in East and West—Taiwan, New York, London, and Hong Kong. After twenty-six years of training with Grandmaster K. H. Chu (London), he was confirmed in 2002 as a 6th-generation master in the Yang-family style. In 1980, he founded the first German Taiji school in Frankfurt, the Taiji Academy, School of Inner Power. Besides teaching, he publishes books and essays and produces educational films (www.tao4me.de)

Having studied musicology at a young age, he also has professional voice training. Music and singing are important parts of his life, as is further research into Taiji, to which he has increasingly devoted himself since discovering particular breathing types.

His books include *AtemtypTaiji: Lehrbuch für lunare Einatmer* (tredition, 2022); *AtemtypTaiji: Lehrbuch für solare Ausatmer* (tredition, 2022); *Das Qi verwurzeln: Qigong und Atemtypen* (Kristkeitz, 2020); *Taiji: Grundlagen einer fernöstlichen Bewegungskunst* (Shaker, 2017); with Volker Brauner & Alexander Zock, *Taiji: Atemenergetik und Biomechanik* (Shaker, 2016); with Judith Hechler, *Innere Kraft durch AtemtypQigong* (Theseus, 2009).

The Authors / 155

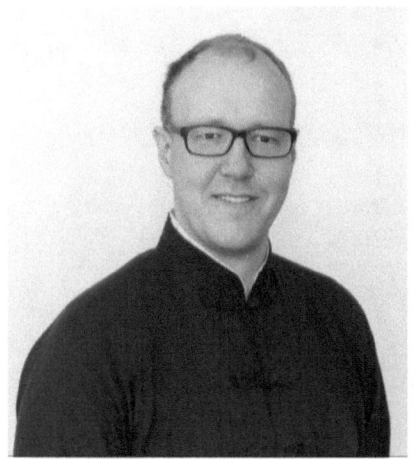

Emanuel Seitz (b. 1985) works as a freelance philosopher and translator in Bad Kreuznach. He studied philosophy, archaeology, history, and Indo-European linguistics in Rome, Freiburg, and Frankfurt, and received his doctorate from the University of Amsterdam. He has practiced Taiji with Frieder Anders since 2018 and is currently in his first year of teacher training. His most recent publication is *List and Form: On Prudence* (Klostermann, 2019) and a translation of Aristophanes' *Clouds* (Munich, 2022).

Index

abdomen: and breath, 31, 81-84; essence in, 126; and gravity, 116, 121-23; *qi* in, 133
Ackermann, Daniel, 105-06
acupuncture, points, 85-87, 90
aerobics, *see* sports
Afrika Korps, 132
aggression, 7, 56-60, 93, 121
Aikido, 41
alchemy: 8-9, 87, internal, 126
Alexander, Fredrick Matthias, 78
aliveness, 135-36, 138
alphorn, 80-81
alternation, see yin and yang
Anders, Frieder, 22, 91, 100-10
anti-aging, 8-10, 37; see also nourishing life
Apollo, 109
archery, 130
Aristotle, 34
arms: extended, 81-83; movements of, 45, 49, 90-91, 116-18, 122, 124, 133-34; muscles of, 69-70, 129; pain in 62, 65; and *qi*, 47, 129; as weapons, 16, 94, 115; *see also* elbows
Art of War, 59
Arte (TV channel), 88
artificiality, 27, 68, 116, 123, 137-38
Ärzteblatt, 62
Astaire, Fred, 75-76
attack, *see* opponent
attention: to flow, 5, 145; and power, 15, 45, 137; and qi, 38, 69, 120, 126, 133-34; and stiffness, 68, 123
authenticity, 28-29
authority, of master, 26, 28-29
Bacon, Francis, 140
balance, 3, 45, 92-93, 104, 118-19, 124, 131, 138
Basho, 28
battery, as metaphor, 85, 135-36

Bauer, Manfred, 101-02
Bauer, Wolfgang, 8-9
Beijing, 20, 98
belief, vs. practice, 144
bellows, as metaphor, 113, 119, 144
Bhutan, 46
Big Five, 101
Blood and Love, 92
Bodhidharma, 110
body: acceptance of, 35; alignment of, 78, 129; awareness of, 10; axis of, 16, 55, 68, 113, 116, 123-24;; and breath, 32-33, 65-66, 81-82; control of, 5, 34; directions of, 123; diseases of, 63; and hands, 69-71; habits, 133; having vs. being, 5-6, 35, 88; health, 114; joints in, 51-52; life energy in, 150; limits of, 47-48; as mechanism, 4-5, 34, 85, 116, 141; and mind, 106; as microcosm, 67, 84, 115, 131; opening of, 129; as organism, 4-5; pain in, 62-63, 67, 81, 110, 130; pillar of, 68, 91-92; posture, 121-23; in practice, 31; pressure, 130; rooting of, 10, 27, 32, 43, 47, 53-55, 76, 98, 121-23, 136; and spirals, 115; and spirit, 45; techniques of, 78; as weapon, 114; weight of, 7; as wheel, 116-17
Böhm, Annett, 81
Bohr, Niels, 5
boxing, 128
Boyd, Robert, 27
brain: and action, 50; and hands, 69-74
breathing types: 073-94, 132-34; definition of, 32-33; exhalers, 134; and exertion, 74-75; experience of, 27, 100; and hand positions, 72; and head, 91; inhalers, 133-34; in lineage, 26; natural,

81-82; and sitting, 64-66; and standing, 54-55
Brecht, Bertold, 142
Buber, Martin, 148
Buddha, 46, 56
Buddhism, 64, 126, 142
buffalo, 59-60
car, as metaphor, 85
centeredness, see body, axis of
change, 30-31, 110, 139-40, 147
chaos, 140
Chen style, 17
Chen Weiming, 13, 134
Chen, William, 11
children, 23, 60, 62, 73-74, 88, 117, 122, 133-36
Chongxu zhenjing, 143
Christ, 82
Chu Gin-Soon, 27
Chu King-Hong, 12-13, 15, 17, 22, 26-29, 35, 39, 41, 70, 76-77, 85, 110, 133
Cirsi, Sibel, 100-01
cocks, fighting, 147
coffee-maker, as metaphor, 85-87
complementarity, 3, 5-6, 30, 117, 140, 148-49
Confucianism, 33, 39, 84, 121, 148
Confucius, 32-33, 143
consciousness, 120
consciousness, and drugs, 88-89
consciousness, development of, 109
consciousness, expansion of, 87-89
Cook Ding, 147
Coubertin, Baron de, 47
creation, 139-40
crucifixion, 82
Cultural Revolution, 19
Dahlke, Rüdiger, 92-93
daily life: change in 030-31, 43-44; goals in, 137-38; giving in, 50; and perfection, 144; practice in, 96, 138; of sages, 138, 145; sedentary, 63-64; vacation from, 44
Dao, 113-14, 139-40
Daodejing, 6, 58, 64, 95, 113, 119, 126, 141-42, 144-46, 148, 150

Daoism, 30, 39, 58, 95, 113-16, 121, 126, 135-36
Daoist Canon, 143-44
Das Chinesische Schattenboxen: Tai Chi, 102
Das Qi verwurzeln, 71
Daumen-Yoga für das Gehirn, 69
Day of the Dead, 90
de Gray, Aubrey, 8
de, 136
death: and birth, 138; and change, 30; for immortals, 114; and life, 117; right to, 96; and stress, 36-37
Deecke, Lüder, 49
Delphi, 109
Der Spiegel, 88
Descartes, René, 34, 47, 126
desires, see emotions
destiny, 68, 83, `35-38, 146-47, 150
dew on grass, as metaphor, 99
diamond, 90-91
diaphragm, 32, 65-66, 74, 82-86
dietary practice, 9, 63, 133, 137
Ding, John, 27
disease, 63, 67, 69, 96, 110, 133, 135, 138-41, 147
disease, in back, 66-68
Dong Yingjie, 11, 16
double helix, 53, 115
dualism, 5, 126, 149-50
Dürckheim, Karlfried Graf, 6, 11, 107
dynamics, 34
dynamics: body, 129; and change, 31, 95, 139, 141; of *qi*, 34-35, 118-19; see also spirals, yin and yang
Dzogchen, 109
earth, grounding in, 53; see also rooting
Easter Bunny, 21, 23, 27
ecstasy, 88-89
Eight Immortals, 9
elasticity, 94, 115, 124, 130
elbows, 51-53; see also arms
Elias, Norbert, 47
elixir fields, 85-87, 91, 122, 126, 134
emotions, 10, 35-38, 58-59, 119, 121, 145

emptiness, 13, 113, 117-20, 135, 144-46, 150
ergonomics, 63
ethics, and *qi*, 95
Feldenkrais, Moshe, 78, 123-25, 130
Fengshui, 137
fibromyalgia, 62
fire, and diamond, 90
fish, as inner power, 27
fishing, as metaphor, 24-25
Five Arts, 42
flow: 5-6, 30-31, 113; of consciousness, 89; of *qi*, 48, 127; and stagnation, 149
force: external, 14-15, 19, 50-51, 114, 128; opposing, 118; patterns of, 3-4; vs. Power, 49; raw, 126-28, 132; of water, 6-7; *see also* inner power, muscles
microcosmic orbit, 132
forces: interplay of, 146; types of, 141
formlessness, 30, 139-41
Frankfurt, 11, 15, 35, 102
Frautschi, Fritz, 80-81
friendliness, 58-59
Frisch, Max 11
Fu Zhongwen, 19-20
Gan Xiaotian, 12
gancui, 13-14
gancui, 134
gardener, as metaphor, 137
Gate of Life/Destiny: 068, 83-87, 91, 133-34; Qigong, 71, 84
Gautier, Théophile, 80
Ge Hong, 8
Gerhardt, Paul, 37
Glaser, Volkmar, 127, 130
Goethe, Johann Wolfgang von, 28
Gongfu, 114, 122
governance, 143
gravity, 121-22, 124
Great Ultimate, 3, 17, 84, 148
Greb, Hans-Peter, 78-79
Gruen, Arno, 93
Guo Xiang, 143
Guodian, 143
Hagena, Charlotte, 74-75, 133

Hagena, Christian, 81
hands, 69-71
Hao Yue-Rue, 66
happiness, 9, 42-44, 104, 109
harmony: cosmic 67, 115, 118-19, 131, 138, 149-50; inner, 3, 121, 141
Hartung, Marion, 104-05
Hasegawa, Yoshiya, 69
Hauskeller, Michael, 48
health, definition of, 43
heart: 35-38, 60; and body, 48; as center, 116; empty, 121; and *qi*, 136; *see also* mind
heaven: and earth, 16, 53, 55, 67-68, 78, 95, 114, 116-17, 121-22, 124-25, 144, 158; salvation in, 138
Heavenly Pass, 68, 86, 91
hedonism, 39
hemispheres, 73-74
Heraclitus, 31
hermits, 9
Hess, Rudolf, 59
hexagrams, 30-31
Höhn, Wolfgang, 11-12, 19, 69
Holmes, Oliver Wendell, 41
Honey, Christian, 8
Hong Kong, 19, 23, 41
Huainanzi, 3
humunculus, 70
Hundred Meeting, 68, 86, 91
Hüther, Gerald, 36-37
I Vow to Attain Eternal Youth, 37
Iceland, 90
immediacy, 46, 56
immortal embryo, 88
immortality, 8-10, 114, 142
immortals, 136, 145, 150-51
improvisations, 49
impulse, 49-50, 56, 58, 88, 122, 127-28
India, 89
infinity, 15, 48, 56, 99, 114-15, 125
inner power: 6-7, 85-97, 126-34; and authenticity, 29; and breath, 74; definition of, 13-15; growth of, 124
inner power, *jin*, 127; effortless, 130; and mind, 128; painless, 118; path

to, 107-08; reservoir of, 114-15; testing of, 50; transmission of, 25-26; and unity, 121
intention, 16, 35, 46-47, 122-23, 126-27; energy, power, 16, 50, 119, 126,, 130
International Tai Chi Chuan Association, 14, 23
inversions, 121
Ip Taitak, 27
Jaack, Sven Joachim, 56
Judo, 42
Jullien, François, 61, 120
Jungle Camp, 47
Kästner, Erich, 63
Kelly, Gene, 75-76
Kessler, Johannes, 37
kidneys, pillars of, 84, 86
King, Warrior, Magician, Lover, 92
Kinoshita, 107
kite-flying, 17
Kleist, Heinrich von, 88, 127
Kornhuber, Hans Helmut, 49
Korycik, Andreas, 104-05
Kroggel, Uwe, 108
Lagemann, Brigitte, 103-04
Lahm, Philip, 63
Laozi, 142
Larsen, Christian, 78
learning styles, 33
Lee, Bruce, 18
left-handers, 73-74
Lessmann, Dardo, 99
leverage, 59-60
Levine, James, 63-64
Li Er, 142
Libet, Benjamin, 50
Liezi, 143
limpness, 69-70, 121, 129-30, 132, 135
longevity techniques, 9, 133, 137
Louguatai Monastery, 142
Luk, Charles, 32
lungs: and breathing, 32, 83m 131-32, 134; meridian, 71
Luserke, Martin, 92
manipura, 85
Mars and Venus, 92-93

martial arts, 16-17, 19, 23, 46, 93, 101, 114-15, 124, 128, 132
master-disciple relationship, 25-29, 32, 98, 100-10, 133
Mawangdui, 142
medicine: Chinese, 38, 85, 127, 141; Western, 18, 35, 37, 62-72, 85, 88-89, 96, 129; *see also* science
meditation, 32, 38, 64, 127, 145
Mencius, 35, 94-97, 119-20
meridians, 127, 129
Merkel, Angela, 90
Messner, Reinhold, 53
metaphysics, 114
Middle Ages, 90
middle path, 96
military, *see* strategy
mind: and body, 48-50, 94, 106, 121, 126-28; and breath, 15-16; empty, 37, 119, 147; fasting of, 38-39, 145; and inner power, 52, 128, 136; and matter, 34; monkey, 105, 120; and movement, 5, 25, 45, 56; persistence of, 130; thinking, 30, 43, 137;
mindfulness, 69, 88, 103, 107
mingmen, see Gate of Life
Mitteldeutscher Rundfunk, 81
Moegling, Klaus, 62
Möller, Katja, 107-08
moon, and finger, 48-49
Morgenstern, Christian, 44
mother, as metaphor, 137
Mount Wudang, 21, 114
movement, 123-25
movement: and breathing types, 76, 131-33; from core, 116; as Dao, 139; calm, 127; external, 27; extreme, 129; micro, 7; relaxed, 122; and spine, 116; spiral, 51-53; *see also* flow
mudras, 72
Mühlhausen, orinna, 43
muscles: in hands, 70-71; respiratory, 75; strength of, 7, 16, 34, 47, 49-50, 65, 84, 94, 114-15, 117, 122, 125, 127-28, 146
music, 80-81, 115-16, 132

mysticism, 8
namelessness, 140-41
Nanhua zhenjing, 143
nature, and Daoism, 140
Nazis, 59
Neijing tu, 98
neurology, 127
New China, 20
New York, 11, 49, 89
Non-Ultimate, 148
nonaction, 56-57, 95-97, 117, 119-21, 143, 146-47
nonbeing, 113, 119, 139-40, 144-45, 148
nose rings, 59-60
nourishing life, 8-9, 39, 136038, 145, 150
Novel *1984*, 29
Novum Organon, 140
obedience, 23, 140
Ocean of Qi, 123
Oedipus, 23
Old Authentic Yang Style, 29
Old Man and the Sea, 24-25
Olympics, 47
opponent, *see* push-hands, victory
opposites: alternation of, 30, 65, 93, 117, 149; unity of, 3-6; *see also* complementarity, yin and yang
organs, 32, 38, 70, 81, 141
origin: cosmic, 53, 139-40; of *qi*, 83-84, 126; return to, 31, 37, 88, 144-45, 150
Orwell, George, 29
Osho, 89
ox-herding, 59-60
pain in combat, 13
pain, in sparring, 15, 17, 30, 42, 47, 59, 125, 128
pandemic, 37
pantheon, 136
Paul, Jean, 42
Peking form, 18
pelvis, 54, 75-76, 80, 134; and breathing, 83-84, 123
Penfield, Wilder, 70
People's Republic, 18, 21
perfected, 136, 139, 145, 150

philosophy, 30-31, 39, 94-95, 114, 126, 135-36, 139-40, 142-44, 149
physical therapy, 67
physics, 115
Picabia, Francis, 51
Picasso, 35
Pietschmann, Herbert, 34-35, 43
pillar: in kidneys, 84, 86; of the person, 68, 91-92
pore breathing, 131
Postman, Neil, 63
posture: and breath, 81-82; and breathing types, 54, 133; and diamond, 91-92; seated, 63-64
potency, 136
progress, 104, 122
psychology, 113
pulse, 44-45, 132
puppets, 127
push-hands, 6-7, 13-15, 42, 52, 56-60, 115-18, 120, 122, 124
qi: in body, 141; cultivation of, 35, 126; circulation of, 10, 116, 119, 122, 129, 131, 141, 149; definition of, 131; flood-like, 94-95; force of, 136; from feet, 42, 129; happy, 39-40, 42-44, 99, 110, 128; as inner fire, 90; movements of, 123, 149-50; in practice, 147
Qigong, 8, 10, 35, 54, 66-70, 96, 102-03, 110, 119, 126
quantum physics, 5
Rajneesh, 89
Reinartz, Stefan, 46
relaxation, 3, 43-44, 104, 107, 122
Renaissance, 34
Right against Right, 59
righteousness, 95-96
Rilke, Rainer Maria, 150
Rolf, Ida, 78
Romans, 82
Roosevelt, Franklin D., 66
runes, 90
sages, 136, 138, 145, 149-51
salmon, as metaphor, 35-37
Schopenhauer, Arthur, 49

162 / Index

Schubert, Helmut, 23
science, 4, 8, 34, 43, 62, 67, 140
scriptures, 144
secrecy, in lineages, 27
Secrets of Chinese Meditation, 32
self: 113; awareness, 33; cultivation, 8-10, 34, 38, 93, 149-50; healing, 37, 96; knowledge, 109; optimization, 33-34; perception, 108; preservation, 58, 124; realization, 99; refinement, 136
senses, withdrawal of, 145
serenity, 3, 9, 39, 96, 114, 123
Seven Sages of the Bamboo Grove, 119
Shaolin Monastery, 110, 128
Shi Ming, 20
Siao Weijia, 20
sitting, 63-64
skills, 61, 93, 147
sky, reaching for, 53
sleep, 94, 97
Smullyan, Raymond M., 58
Snake: 114, 130; Style, 27, 77
soccer, 45-46
solar, vs. lunar 55, 74, 79, 100, 103, 133-34
Song, simpleton of, 95
space: vs. Body, 48; empty, 119
speech, and handedness, 74
spine, 67, 116
spirals, 115-16, 118, 125, 134
spirit: spirit, and consciousness,
spirit, and Dao, 147; guiding, 126-27; and immortality, 8-9, 114, 136-147, 150; and movement, 31, 45, 102, 128; nourishing of, 8; people, 135, 151; as spark, 85, 87; of Taiji, 23, 41, 47, 94, 125;
Splett, Beate, 81
spontaneity, 16, 49, 51, 56-57, 88, 119, 127, 136, 154, 147
sports: 04, 33-34, 37, 114-15, 122, 126, 128; and breathing types, 74-75; and games, 41-42; soccer, 45-46

sprouts, pulling of, 95-96
steel, 128
stillnesss, 45
strategy, 59-61, 114, 119-21, 139, 141
strength: and leverage, 60; team, 46; *see also* muscle
stress, 36-37, 47, 94, 108
Stroh, Thomas 106-07
Süddeutsche Zeitung, 66-67
Sunzi, 59
superstition, 18
Switzerland, 12, 20, 80
symphony, 115-16, 146
Tai Chi im Test der Wissenschaft, 62
Tai Chi Kineo, 106
Taiji: Academy, 56, 62, 75, 78-79, 85-86, 99, 102, 105; classics, 15, 92, 94, 127, 129; definition of, 4; development of, 29; history of, 16-20, 25; internal, 12-13, 15-17, 25, 37, 46, -50, 53-54, 105, 114-17, 119, 122, 125, 129, 131-32; name, 4; as play, 41-42; Ruyi style, 20; for show, 18-19; spirituality, in, 94; styles of, 16-17; symbol, 3, 117, 148-49
Taijitu, 3, 148
Taipei, 12
Taiyi jinhua zongzhi, 144
Tang dynasty, 121
Tao: The Watercourse Way, 6
teachers: quality of, 27-29; ranks of, 100
team strength, 46
Ten Basic Principles, 66, 92, 94
tension: good, 127; muscle, 50, 114, 129, 125, 132; tonic, 130
terlusollogy, 74, 81
theater, 49, 89, 92
therapy, physical, 129
third eye, 88
three treasures, 126, 150
thumbs, 69-71
tiger claw, 16
tiger mouth, 71
time, cyclical, 31
training systems, 17-18
transmission, *see* lineage

tree: becoming of, 49; growth of, 53; in martial arts, 16; rooted, 43; standing like, 124; as symbol, 9; uselessness of, 136
triangle, 71, 91-92
tripod position, 48, 65
Tuscany, 100
Über den Prozess der Zivilisation, 47
unity, 5, 56, 89, 126, 139, 140, 149, 150
Unschuld, Paul, 38
uprightness, 16, 26, 49, 53-55, 64-68, 76, 78, 115-18, 121-27
uprooting, 15, 42, 47, 50, 52, 58, 50, 118, 124, 128, 133-34, 147
US, 89, 102
uselessness, 138, 144
Valery, Paul, 43
valley, as metaphor, 113
vessel, as metaphor, 144-45
victory, 59-60, 93, 116-18, 126, 132, 144, 146
videos, and breathing types, 76
virtue, 136
vitality, 15, 35, 58, 84, 135-37, 150
voice training, 12, 75, 133
volition, *see* will
Vorpahl, Klaus, 98
walking, 55, 79
Wang Bi, 142
Wang Peisheng, 19
Wang Yennian, 12
Wang Yongquan, 20
Wang, Henry, 12
Warum, 107
water, as metaphor, 6-7, 131, 142, 146; *see also* weak
Watts, Alan, 6
We Amuse Ourselves to Death, 63
weak: vs. Hard, 146-47; points, 60; soft and, 6-7, 16, 58-59, 65, 141
weakness, of external practice, 137-38
weapons, in Taiji, 105
Weffer, Rainer, 109-10
Western culture, 31
Western medicine, 34

wheel, as metaphor, 113, 116-17, 121, 134, 144-45, 146
White Cloud Monastery, 98
Whitehead, alfred North, 78
Wikipedia, 65
Wilde, Oscar, 75
Wilk, Erich, 74, 132-33
will power, 81
Wippermann, Peter, 43
Wolfseck, Wolf von, 92
Wu style, 19, 66
Wu Yuxiang, 38, 94, 127
Wunsiedel, 59
Xingming guizhi, 144
Yang Chengfu, 13, 17, 19, 21,22, 25, 28, 44-45, 66, 91-92, 94,
Yang Jianhou, 20, 22
Yang Luchan, 21-22, 30
Yang Ma Lee, 27
Yang Shouzhong, 19, 21-23, 25, 77, 133
Yang Zhendou, 25
Yang Zhenguo, 25
Yang Zhenyi, 25
Yang Zhu, 38-39
Yi Xingzi, 147
Yijing, 3, 30-31, 148
yin and yang: 03-5, 44-045, 72, 114, 117-18, 121, 123, 131-32, 134, 141; attributes of, 150; definition of, 140; in muscles, 129; in Taiji symbol, 148-49
Yin Xi, 142
Yin Yang Form, 117
Yongquan Study Association, 20
YouTube, 20, 25, 27
Zen, 64, 99, 107, 109, 130
Zhang Sanfeng, 21, 114
Zhang Zhan, 143
Zheng Manqing, 11-12, 42
Zhongnan mountains, 142
Zhou Dunyi, 148
Zhou dynasty, 142
Zhu Huaiyuan, 20
Zhuangzi, 24, 132, 135, 136, 138, 143, 145, 147, 151

www.ingramcontent.com/pod-product-compliance
Lightning Source LLC
Chambersburg PA
CBHW032026230426
43671CB00005B/219